D0019923

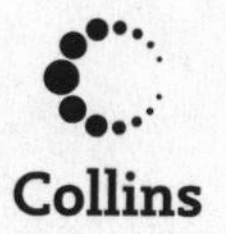
Collins

THE METABOLISM BOOSTING DIET

THE METABOLISM BOOSTING DIET

BURN FAT, BALANCE HORMONES AND LOSE WEIGHT FOR LIFE

DR. JOEY SHULMAN

D.C., REGISTERED NUTRITIONIST

The Metabolism Boosting Diet

Published by Collins, an imprint of HarperCollins Publishers Ltd

First Edition

The Nutrition Facts Table. Health Canada, 2008.
Reproduced with the permission of the Minister of Health, 2011.

HarperCollins Publishers Ltd
2 Bloor Street East, 20th Floor
Toronto, Ontario, Canada
M4W 1A8

www.harpercollins.ca

Library and Archives Canada Cataloguing in Publication
information is available upon request

ISBN 978-1-44340-112-8

Printed and bound in the United States
9 8 7 6 5 4 3 2 1

To Randy, Jonah bear and Faith Ella—my three loves
We are having the "best good" times

And . . . this one's for you, biddy—I could not walk
this journey without you

A million will I's #5 . . . a million will I's

CONTENTS

Appendices

ACKNOWLEDGEMENTS

American publisher Katharine Graham, who once presided over the *Washington Post*, has been quoted as saying, "To love what you do and feel that it matters—how could anything be more fun?" This is precisely how I feel about nutrition, weight loss and writing. I still pinch myself each and every day that I am able to publish my beliefs and passion for nutrition and natural health care and share them with you.

There are a few core people who need acknowledgement in helping this book come to be. First and foremost, thank you to my sister, Laina, for her countless hours of working with me on this project. There were many times when she was able to put into words what I could not and therefore, part of her essence is within the context of these pages. A million thank yous, Lain, for all that you do.

I also must thank each and every weight loss client I have worked with over the years. It has been my sincere pleasure and greatest joy to help you lose the weight, get healthier, hear your stories and learn from you. Many of your experiences, successes, trials and accomplishments are woven within the pages of this book. All of you are examples of what is possible.

To the staff and nutritionists at Shulman Weight Loss Clinic, thank you. You make a difference in the lives of so many people looking to lose the weight . . . and to live their lives.

To Brad Wilson at HarperCollins and my agent, Rick Broadhead, thank you for the encouragement and support that allowed me to stick to the sincerity of my vision.

To the Shulman clan—love to the moon and beyond. Mom and Dad—you are the glue and we adore you. May we have many more "Windermere-like" memories.

To Jonah and Faith Ella—my two heart songs. Jonah, when G-d gave out joy, you truly got a double dose. You make Daddy and me laugh each and every day. Little Faith—oh how we waited for you, sweet one. Your sparkly eyes are very familiar and your bubbly spirit brings so much to our lives.

To my *besheret*, Randy. You help me daily with my worrying ways and never seem to grow weary of my questions. I love you in every way and it keeps getting stronger. May the good times we are having continue always. When I am with you, I am home.

INTRODUCTION

A grand adventure is about to begin.
—Winnie the Pooh

WHY DID I WRITE THIS BOOK?

Even as a five-time author, each time I sit down to pen a book, I experience a degree of excitement and nervousness about beginning a new project. Not only was writing *The Metabolism Boosting Diet* incredibly exciting for me, but it was a distinctively unique experience. Before writing the book, I had been blessed to work with thousands of men, women and teens on their weight loss journey. Seeing their dramatic health improvements along with their significant weight loss success—from 15 to 100 pounds or more—has been the most rewarding work of my life. Every time I witness a new client following the system, losing the weight and feeling better, I comment to my clinic director that it is as though they have found their shine once again. As their health improves and their weight goes down, their shoulders go back, their skin clears, their energy soars, and their surge in confidence can be felt and seen. The layers of heaviness of poor health and excess weight that they first walked into the clinic with are gone, and the "lightness" of optimal health and vitality gets the chance to shine through.

Although seeing the weight melt off my clients is thrilling and we celebrate each and every pound and inch gone, there is more to this process than just the number on the scale or tape measure. Why? *Because health is the first wealth.* As my client Marianna, a recent cancer survivor, said through tears, "Joey, this is about far more than just fitting into my jeans." While Marianna acknowledged that losing the weight and dropping sizes felt great, she was aware of something even bigger taking place. She was using her food and dietary intake as a powerful preventative approach to disease and, as she put it, it was "one of her greatest tools for living her best life."

Within these pages, and with the permission of my clients, I share a number of their stories and pictures with you. Whether it is the mother of five young children, the professional who was just dumped by her boyfriend, the post-menopausal woman who told me she would never lose weight, or the CEO of a Fortune 500 company, my goal is to show you that they . . . are you. It does not matter what you do for a living, how much weight you have to lose or what age you are—I assure you, you can and will do this.

After watching the most amazing transformations, what I know for sure is that using optimal nutrition as the platform to propel your life to a higher level is a guaranteed path. As you will discover and see in the pages of this book, the health and life changes that begin by simply changing your food and following the Metabolism Boosting Diet are nothing short of breathtaking.

And now it's time for you to put yourself on your own to-do list and take control of your health with food. I assure you, when you eat better, you feel better and do better each and every time.

Let's begin!

EVERY JOURNEY BEGINS WITH JUST ONE STEP

Let's be honest, shall we? Weight loss is about much more than counting carbohydrates, limiting calories or following weekly weigh-ins. In truth, to lose the weight for life and for your results to stick, you must change nutritionally, physically and emotionally. If the change is not permanent and the plan is not sound and achievable, all results will be temporary. The plan has to fit you and your metabolism to provide lifelong results.

After working in the weight loss world for over a decade, I have seen it all. I have also been witness to the fact that things fall off track and need to be steered back to what works. For example, I regularly see clients who, before implementing the Metabolism Boosting Diet, have fallen into diet traps—eating 500 to 600 calories a day, restricting their intake of all fats, drinking smoothies for meals, ordering food by mail, or dropping all forms of carbohydrates. In short, whatever promises to work, they will do it. Although these unbalanced approaches may trigger some weight loss in the beginning stages, in the long run they typically conk out your metabolism's engine, making future weight loss attempts even harder and more frustrating. On a deeper level, these types of quick-fix dietary approaches create further damage to your relationship with food and move you even farther from hitting your long-term health and weight loss goals. Drained of energy—and often money—and disappointed by their failed attempt, most people either move on to the next diet that seems to offer the answer or give up entirely.

It's time to end the insanity that is occurring in the weight loss world.

WE ARE INDEED MUCH MORE THAN WHAT WE EAT

Nutritional pioneer Adelle Davis has been quoted as saying, "We are indeed much more than what we eat, but what we eat can help us to become much more than who we are." In other words, of course you are greater than the burger you had at lunch or the pasta you ate at dinner; however, the food you eat will be the foundation that helps the "best you" to flourish. When you eat better, you feel better and therefore can do better.

On a first visit with weight loss clients, I listen carefully to the terminology they use to describe their current state of health and how they are feeling. *Stuffed, bloated, uncomfortable, out of control, depressed* and *sluggish* are words I often hear. How can you possibly be the best at your job as a parent, partner or sibling when so much of your energy is tied up with your food, your weight and your body image? Wouldn't it be liberating to finally free up that energy and shift to a stage that is far healthier and more productive? The good news is you can!

Before prescribing a weight loss program to any of my clients, I ask two fundamental questions:

1. How many times a day do you think about your weight?
2. On a scale of zero to 10, how much does your weight affect your mood on a daily basis? (Zero means it does not affect your mood; 10 means it dramatically affects it.)

These questions are integral to the Metabolism Boosting Diet because they highlight how being overweight affects you on so many levels. The majority of my weight loss clients initially report thinking of their weight 3 or more times per day and rank the effect on their mood as 8 or higher. Now ask yourself these same questions. If you think of your weight more than 2 or 3 times a day and you rank the effect your weight has on your mood as 7 or higher—well, that is far too much energy for you to waste and it is time to stop. It is time to shift to a dietary approach that promotes health, balance and long-term sustainable results.

Along this journey we are about to take together, I encourage you to become aware of your eating patterns and to be compassionate with yourself. Since approximately 66% of Canadians currently struggle with their weight, I assure you, you are not alone. I also want you to know that you are not weak or lacking in willpower. However, chances are, due to a variety of reasons that will be determined as we go along, there are factors (stress, lack of sleep, hormonal imbalances, yo-yo dieting, emotional or nighttime eating) that have burnt out or slowed down your metabolism, making you gain unwanted weight. Do not panic: in this book you will learn the steps you need to take to flick on your metabolic switch so that you can lose the weight for good.

WHAT IS THE ANSWER TO THE WEIGHT LOSS RIDDLE?

To take weight off for life, you must attack the problem on two levels: physical and emotional. This process is actually quite simple and will provide you with far more control over your food choices and behaviours than you have ever had. You will find that, once you have successfully completed the Metabolism Boosting Diet, you will enjoy food more than ever before and will feel totally satiated. Your excess weight will no longer be the "monkey on your shoulder" you need to deal with, and you'll enjoy all situations, from socializing and eating out on the weekends to holidays and travelling, without weight gain or food guilt. Not only will you love the food you are eating but you will also love the new body, energy and look you have been able to easily obtain. I frequently remind my clients that, unlike addictive substances (alcohol, drugs, cigarettes), we cannot eliminate food from our life completely. Thus, we must make peace with our food so we can once again enjoy all the goodness and joy it has to offer.

DECLUTTER AND FIND YOUR *WHY*

Unlike most other diets, your journey on the Metabolism Boosting Diet begins with a decluttering process. In addition to getting all the unhealthy foods out of your home, it's important to get rid of, at a deeper level, all the clutter or "noise" that's coming to you from the weight loss world. All too often, weight loss seekers are lured by lofty promises of overly rapid weight loss results ("30 pounds in 2 months!"), magic bullets, surgeries or treatments that supposedly suck out the fat. Not only can these approaches be frustrating, offering short-lived results, but they can also damage and slow down your metabolism. As a starting point for any weight loss program, you must ask yourself, *Can I see myself following a version of this program in 5 years' time?* If the answer is no, don't do it. If the program doesn't entail a permanent shift that fits into your life and is simple to follow, it will be a frustrating exercise in futility. In other words, if the change in dietary behaviour is overly restrictive—involving counting points, limiting bites, restricting calories and taking pills, for example—it will ultimately be short-lived, and so too will be the weight loss results.

When it comes to diet and food changes, an integral step in the shift toward long-lasting success is to connect to your *why*. Determining your *why* is a simple and quick process that is explained in more detail in Chapter 2. While it may sound a little out there, it's actually a strategy followed by the most successful companies in the world. The Apple company, for instance, became the success it is today by determining its *why* from the outset. Apple's *why* was to put the ease of technology in our hands (as I type on my beloved Apple computer, I assure you, it did it!). Once Apple determined its *why*, the company implemented its *do* and enjoyed the results. Why should weight loss be any different? Once you determine your *why*, you'll learn the *do* (the principles to boost metabolism and burn fat at an effective rate for the long term) and then you will enjoy the results: long-term weight loss success. The *why* will be the platform of inspiration and motivation to ensure you lose the weight and maintain the results for life.

What I know for sure, after working with thousands of people who have successfully lost weight, is that the clients who take the extra weight off and keep it off typically start the process by discovering their *why*.

It does not matter if you have 15, 50 or 100 pounds to lose—you can and you will. The fact that you are reading this means that you are craving more balance, more peace and greater vitality from the food you eat. This is always the first and most important part of the process.

BOOSTING YOUR METABOLISM . . . AT ANY AGE AND ANY STAGE

The rate at which people burn fat, lose weight and boost their metabolism is quite different from individual to individual. This is one of the many reasons why I do not practice cookie-cutter or one-size-fits-all weight loss or recommend such approaches. For example, one woman may be post-menopausal and on a medication that alters her metabolic engine, such as thyroid medication, whereas another woman is under high levels of stress and not sleeping at night. Everyone's metabolism is unique and has different influencing factors, such as age, hormonal health, genetic history, stress and activity level. This is why person A will easily lose 5 pounds each and every week, while person B may lose 1 to 2 pounds per week. After closely following clients' metabolic patterns over the years, I have developed a unique system that can accurately identify the state of your metabolism and thereby match you with a detailed nutritional and lifestyle plan to boost your metabolic rate and weight loss potential to its maximum level. As you will soon discover, this system encompasses much more than just the food on your plate. It's a system designed to "hit it out of the park" on all weight loss fronts and create lifelong changes.

In Part III, you will find the plan—that is, the *do* part. After completing the Metabolic ID Questionnaire in Chapter 6 (which takes into account your hormonal status, age, dieting history, physical activity levels and emotional relationship with food), you will be assigned a personal plan that will stabilize your blood sugars, balance your hormones, boost your metabolism and re-establish your relationship with food. Your daily food structure, meal plans, recipes and grocery shopping list—as well as effective techniques to break cravings and plateaus—will all be detailed for you. Once you have the Metabolism Boosting Diet tools mastered and in your back pocket, you can fall off the health wagon (say, at your birthday party, on weekends or on holidays) and simply jump back on at any time. *You* will have the control—not the food or the cravings.

SIMPLIFY, SIMPLIFY, SIMPLIFY

Along with identifying how your metabolism functions, burning fat and reaching your ultimate goal weight, the other focus of the Metabolism Boosting Diet is to make food fun and simple again. Instead of concentrating on what you are going to take out of your diet, the key is to focus on the delicious (and easy-to-prepare) food that you are going to put back into it. Before long, you will find that all my recommendations and suggestions that you follow have become second nature, leading to lifelong habits. By following the simple guidelines in each chapter, you will find you are able to keep yourself at your target weight and you feel energetic, vibrant and spry. Life is so busy and full for all of us—who has time to spend energy on diets and carry excess weight? Let's make food fun, delicious and simple once again!

PART I
THE PREMISE

CHAPTER 1
MAKING IT WORK FOR YOU

Take care of your body. It's the only place you have to live.
—Jim Rohn, author and inspirational speaker

ARE YOU SATISFIED?

I have been practicing yoga with the same teacher for more than 20 years. During the class, the yogi talks us through the poses while discussing issues of emotional and physical health and healing. With over 43 years of teaching experience and thousands of students each year, the yogi shares pearls of wisdom with us every week that fascinate me.

At a recent class, the yogi discussed change and said, "Dissatisfaction is an indication of progress." As soon as he said this, a light bulb went off in my head. Instead of thinking of dissatisfaction as something bad and pushing the feeling away, we should welcome it. In fact, dissatisfaction is one of the most powerful ways our subconscious nudges us to make a change. Whether we want to lose weight, quit smoking or be more patient, when we are feeling some level of dissatisfaction and discontent, it is our inner being gently nudging us to go for more. Call this feeling an intuition or a sign, it doesn't really matter. What matters is that if your level of dissatisfaction leads you to take the action steps to demand more, you will be able to get to where you want to be.

THE "BUT JOEYS"

In order to start fresh, I keep in mind the Latin term *tabula rasa*, which literally translates as "blank slate." Do not focus on past weight loss attempts that have failed or on your journey ahead; just take a deep breath and begin with a clear vision and a clear mind.

For those people wishing to begin anew, I encourage them to first get rid of any mental barriers that may be standing in their way. Such a barrier is often what I call the "But Joey." I find that, in clinic, I hear these two little words a lot, especially when clients are just beginning their weight loss journey.

All of us have trepidations about starting something new or overcoming a hurdle that has been standing in our way. The "But Joeys" are normal—they're common reservations rooted in the fear of, or resistance to, failing with yet another diet. Often we do not believe we have the willpower to start another program, or we feel too overwhelmed by life to take on anything else. In truth, there is always a something that can block you from starting—a social function, a stressful situation at home, work deadlines. However, when other areas in your life are reeling, losing the weight and taking back control of your health helps tremendously. You feel better, stronger, more focused, more patient at home and better able to deal with life's little (or big) punches. Of course, losing the weight is not a cure-all for all the stressors or unwelcome events in your life—but it does help you to maintain a better balance. Once we clear the roadblocks—or the symptoms of "excusitis," as I call it in jest—we can start with gusto.

BUT JOEY, I HAVE A VERY SLOW METABOLISM!

Of all the issues and excuses I hear, this is one of the most common. Regardless of whether their unwanted excess weight is due to age, genetic history, hormonal fluctuations or lack of activity, people commonly blame it on their so-called slow metabolism. So let's deal with this issue of slow metabolism from the get-go.

In essence, everyone has a unique metabolism—some faster than others; however, there are several influencing factors that can boost and improve the potential and functioning of your metabolism. With the proper implementation and integration of the principles outlined in the following pages, you will find that there is no limit to weight loss. Whether the reason for your excess weight is hormonal, emotional, lifestyle or other—you can and will tackle it.

Take for example my client Annie. On our first visit, Annie told me she had been struggling with her weight for more than 5 years. After having a hysterectomy 3 years previously and being on medication since, Annie, at 5 feet 4 inches, was very upset with now weighing in at 170 pounds. Her energy was extremely low (she was beginning to nap throughout the day) and her stress levels were very high, largely due to her excess weight. She had an intense sweet tooth and was routinely eating gelato in the evening once everyone else in the house was asleep as her reward for a hard day.

At our first meeting, my impression was that Annie was quite vulnerable and also nervous about starting the Metabolism Boosting Diet. Like so many others, Annie described her metabolism as very slow and was skeptical about whether her body would respond to the program. Because of her health history and her unsuccessful 5-year fight to lose the weight, she was honest enough with me to say, "Dr. Joey, I don't think this will work." Tired, frustrated and almost ready to give up, Annie had landed in my office only because a friend of hers had been successful on the program. Looking at

Annie's situation, it was obvious what was happening. Her metabolic engine was completely conked out because she was inactive, out of hormonal balance, very stressed and oversecreting cortisol, a stress hormone. She was also eating far too many refined and highly processed sugary treats at night, which were causing her to oversecrete the hormone insulin, which in turn was causing excess fat to be stored in her abdominal region. Annie's patterns of emotional eating (sweets at night when alone) made her feel far from herself. It was definitely time for a change.

I explained to Annie that to correct the problem, we would first have to determine her metabolic ID (type), get her into hormonal and blood sugar balance and implement metabolic-boosting principles. Once she lost the weight, I would teach her how to shift and maintain her results without the fear of gaining back the weight. She hesitantly agreed, and to her credit put her chin to the ground and implemented all the changes I recommended.

Much to Annie's surprise, week by week, she kept on losing weight. Once nervous about starting the program, Annie now reported that she felt her new dietary approach had changed her life. Within a short time, Annie found her shine; she was walking with her shoulders back and her head high, wearing her new skinny jeans, and had a joie de vivre that had certainly been missing on her first visit with me. I am thrilled to report that as I write this, Annie has lost 32 pounds, is down 8 inches around her waist and has an abundant amount of energy. She is vibrant, healthy and eager to continue on her journey. She recently celebrated her health success at her son's bar mitzvah, where she was comfortable enough to have people lift her up and down on a chair during the hora (a celebratory dance). Bravo, Annie!

What Annie says . . .

I still remember vividly the first week when I lost several pounds and wondered how that was possible. I kept getting back on the scale to make sure it was right! I actually could not figure out why it was working, since I couldn't lose weight on my own. I love the changes I have made and the additions to my meals—so simple and easy. I never felt like I was on a diet because I was eating more than before. I was also not measuring and weighing my food. It has been an enlightening journey I did not expect.

BUT JOEY, I'M POST-MENOPAUSAL!

I routinely encounter this "But Joey." And yes, I understand. Half of my practice is post-menopausal, a stage when weight gain tends to occur in the abdominal region. That being said, being peri- or post-menopausal does not have to translate into being overweight. Being in this stage of life will change your Metabolic ID Questionnaire score slightly; the Metabolism Boosting Diet is designed to take this into account. By discovering your metabolic ID, getting into blood sugar and hormonal balance and following the metabolic-boosting plan outlined for you, you can lose the weight no matter what your age. You'll also find that the weight you lose is targeted fat. In other words, when fat is lost in the proper way, it tends to come off those areas you want it to the most—the abdominal region and love handles.

BUT JOEY, I'VE TRIED EVERY DIET IN THE WORLD!

If this is your "But Joey," you must stop being a lifer in the weight loss world. The one thing that the body hates more than carrying around excess weight is gaining and losing it, gaining and losing it. In fact, studies show that gaining and losing weight repetitively can greatly increase your risk for developing heart disease, in addition to slowing down your metabolism's potential.

To break this cycle, we need to go back to that fundamental question, "Can I see myself following a version of this program in 5 years' time?" I always tell my clients that I am not interested in seeing them losing weight temporarily. Why would I be? My name is on the door of my clinic, on all my books—my intention and goal is always to teach the tools to make permanent health and weight loss shifts. My job is to teach you the principles to discover your metabolic ID, to balance your hormones and sugar and to boost your metabolism. And then, once you do that and the weight is gone, how to maintain your weight loss results for life. I am always delighted when I bump into a former weight loss client 2 or 3 years after they implemented the Metabolism Boosting Diet and they give me a smile from ear to ear because they are still at their goal weight. To me, that is true success.

BUT JOEY, I AM AN EMOTIONAL EATER!

Who isn't? I truly believe that, on some level, we are all emotional eaters. Stressed, bored, sad, lonely, even happy—we eat! Let's face it, food is intimately linked with our emotions and how we respond to situations. At some point in our lives, most of us turn to food for a little extra comfort. While emotional eating is not about the food itself, getting into hormonal balance and cutting your cravings will help to calm the "need" to eat sweets. Once you are in a better, more balanced state with food, you can tackle emotional eating and employ strategies for success.

As I mentioned earlier, an integral step to putting an end to emotional eating is discovering your *why,* which you will do in the next chapter. Once you have identified your *why,* you will possess the motivation and inspiration (even when times are tough) to keep you on track. Be patient with yourself—Rome was not built in a day. Food behaviours are often the hardest to change, but as you shift, so will your emotional connection and relationship to food.

BUT JOEY, I HAVE SUCH A SWEET TOOTH!

Ah, the sweet tooth. I know you may feel at this moment that you suffer with sweet tooth syndrome, but I assure you, the need for sweets will break after the first few days on the program. There is a big difference between enjoying sweets and needing or craving them. Most of us enjoy sweet foods; however, a true sugar craving is a chemical reaction that tips us into a pattern of eating that triggers weight gain and continual up-and-down energy cycles. If you are eating to bring energy up, if you feel that 3 p.m. slump, if you feel you *need* to have a cookie instead of simply wanting it or if you tend to binge eat in the midst of an intense craving, chances are you are bouncing around your blood sugars and storing excess weight in your abdominal region. On the Metabolism Boosting Diet, the cravings will be no more. You will be able to eat naturally sweet foods without cravings for unhealthy refined treats.

BUT JOEY, I HAVE NO TIME!

Yes, you do. What you do not have time for is ill health, poor energy, feeling sad or depressed and a lack of self-confidence because of the way you look and feel. I have been fortunate to have worked with extremely successful individuals who run multi-million-dollar companies, raise busy families and are on the proverbial hot seat at all times. From famous musicians and actors to politicians and executives who virtually live at the airport, they made the time to feel better—and so can you.

BUT JOEY, I AM ALREADY A HEALTHY EATER!

If this is the case, I am thrilled. I often find relatively healthy eaters at my clinic. They are well versed on eating whole grains, vegetables, fruits and lean proteins and are open to incorporating more healthy choices into their diet. If you are a healthy eater, this is terrific news and makes the journey we are about to take only easier. You will find that the Metabolism Boosting Diet will pinpoint the appropriate tweaks needed in your diet (portion control, blood sugar balancing and so on) to help you lose your desired weight and feel your very best.

BUT JOEY, IT IS TOO EXPENSIVE!

I never really understood this particular "But Joey." First off, health indeed is the first wealth and comes before everything. Even so, engaging in a healthier lifestyle and losing weight does not have to be much more expensive. Years ago, my husband and I calculated shopping at the "healthy" store versus the "unhealthy" one. The healthier store came in at approximately $22 more for a week's worth of groceries. Keep in mind that on the Metabolism Boosting Diet you will eat nutrient-dense foods filled with flavour, nutrition, healthy fats, whole grains and naturally occurring sugars. A majority of these foods do not have to cost more; you simply need to become aware of how to shop for them and how to prepare them. I also outline helpful ways to cut costs along the way—for example, which foods are more important than others to purchase organic.

In addition to the above list of "But Joeys," there may be other limitations in your life restricting you from taking your health and weight by the reins. I assure you, there is no greater venture than taking the path of health. If you feel something is holding you back, identify your roadblocks so that we can start on the exciting path to feeling like your best self once again.

THE FIVE TRUTHS OF WEIGHT LOSS

This above all: to thine own self be true. —William Shakespeare

Before beginning the Metabolism Boosting Diet, let's identify the five fundamental weight loss truths. These principles are rarely discussed in the conventional weight loss world, rarely marketed or seen on television ads, yet they are truthful and dig a little deeper into the how and why of weight loss—and therefore elicit sustained results.

Feeling overwhelmed? Simply take baby steps. You will notice discernible changes by making every day slightly better than the day before. Drink more water; drop all processed, refined foods or get up and move. Remember, the better it gets, the better it gets!

TRUTH #1: IT IS IMPORTANT TO LOSE WEIGHT WITH DIGNITY, IN A SAFE AND SUSTAINABLE MANNER

During my time in the weight loss world, I have seen a lot of extremes. I have had men and women who were instructed to take 20 or more pills per day, were encouraged to order food by mail or were bullied and yelled at by the doctor supervising their weight loss when they did not lose what was expected of them. I have also seen people go extreme with certain crash diets and experience hair loss, constipation, fatigue and dizziness. One woman in my practice who had taken an extreme high-protein approach failed her life insurance policy exam because her liver enzymes were so elevated she was thought to be an alcoholic, even though she didn't drink alcohol! Rather, her liver enzymes were elevated because of the desperate (and unsafe) measures she was taking to lose weight.

What I have found with both my readers and clients is that it is of the utmost importance to lose weight with dignity and in a safe and sustainable manner. Your health venture should be supported by loved ones (if you choose to share), should be reasonable and sound (based on science) and should enhance, not hinder, your overall energy, lifestyle and confidence levels. The more you learn about the Metabolism Boosting Diet—your personal metabolic ID, blood sugar control, hormonal balance and metabolic-boosting principles—the more you will be empowered by the knowledge to create permanent change.

TRUTH #2: YOU CANNOT BREAK UP WITH FOOD

Among all addictions and dependencies, unhealthy food behaviour is one of the most difficult to change. This is ultimately why so many quick-fix diets fail: they don't encourage you to discover your *why* and make peace with food. Or they urge you to "lose it faster," practice "rapid weight loss" and look like the model on the cover of a magazine overnight. In truth, losing weight is an emotional and physical journey that has to be integrated into new behaviour and thought patterns. Unlike tobacco, alcohol or drugs, food cannot be eliminated from our lives. Therefore, you need to fine-tune your dance with food in order to move forward. Once you have the tools to do this, you are freed and can finally make peace with food.

TRUTH #3: YOU MUST IDENTIFY YOUR TRIGGERS

If you examine your eating patterns, you will surely notice specific times of day or certain situations when you fall off the health wagon. Perhaps you drink a glass of wine too many nights after the kids are asleep, overindulge in the cheese and crackers before dinner or eat sugary candy to bring your energy levels up when experiencing the dreaded 3 p.m. slump. By identifying your triggers, you can bring more awareness to your eating patterns, which will in turn alter your choices. The more awareness you can bring to your eating patterns, the greater success you will have long term. Simply start by identifying the time of day you are triggered to eat and what foods are your go-tos.

TRUTH #4: YOU GOTTA WANNA

As I said in the Introduction, when I ask clients, "On a scale of zero to 10, how much does your weight affect your mood on a daily basis?" the response I get, from all walks of life, is typically 8 or higher. And that's too high! Excess weight and poor health can affect you on many levels—physically, emotionally, spiritually and energetically. However, to make a change, you gotta wanna! The fact that you are reading this book means that you are ready to take the weight off, integrate new behaviours and form a healthier relationship with food. Perhaps you have been burned in the past by false weight loss promises or have struggled with your weight for so many years that you are close to giving up. I implore you, do not give up—you can do it! The wanting is the first brick on your pathway to success. You have already stepped onto it by picking up this book—bravo!

TRUTH #5: FOR A LIFELONG WEIGHT LOSS SHIFT TO OCCUR, YOU MUST BRING MINDFULNESS TO YOUR EATING

A client of mine once said to me, "You can't binge eat and practice mindful eating at the same time." I couldn't agree more. This program will not only teach you principles that will boost your metabolism and put you into hormonal balance with food, it will also teach you methods to eat at a conscious level that will help you to enjoy your food on a deeper level.

Are you ready to begin the Metabolism Boosting Diet? If so, let's move on to Chapter 2 to determine your *why*.

CHAPTER 2
FINDING YOUR *WHY*

Don't ask yourself what the world needs; ask yourself what makes you come alive. And then go and do that. Because what the world needs is people who have come alive.
—Harold Thurman

Weight loss is extremely personal and often an "aha" moment is needed for you to take the initiative and get back control of your health. Consider my client Cara. A very busy mother of three boys who was constantly running from hockey game to hockey game with her kids, Cara was also doing all the bookkeeping for her husband's company as well as continually cooking, cleaning and playing chauffeur to her busy children. Unfortunately, this hectic pace of life left little time for Cara to put herself on her list of people to take care of, and she started to make poor food choices. Like so many others, she started to overeat the wrong foods at night as a reward for her hard day and was resorting to drive-thrus for a quick pick-me-up muffin and coffee during the day. Making poor food choices, tired and inactive, Cara started to gain weight and her cholesterol levels began to rise. Instead of going on medication for her high cholesterol, Cara ended up in my office with 40 pounds to lose.

At our first meeting, Cara told me that she was depressed because she did not fit into any of her clothes. She also refused to buy one to two sizes larger because she felt like that would be giving up. Even though she was desperate to lose the weight and felt quite uncomfortable, Cara was, she confessed, hesitant to start the program. She began to list her many reasons why. She told me she had family coming in from out of town soon, part of her house was being redone and tax season was around the corner, meaning she would be extremely busy. While on some level Cara was ready to change—she booked and then showed up for her appointment, after all—she was also trying to come up with every possible excuse why she could not start. She had thrown up her roadblocks before we had even begun.

To point out her need to commit to change and explore why she had these perceived limitations, I gently asked Cara to use five words or phrases to describe how she was feeling on a daily basis. Her responses were "tired, depressed, out of control, uncomfortable and numb." How could those feelings not evoke an emotion that would initiate change? When it came down to it, Cara admitted that although she wanted to change, she was afraid of failing and did not know if she possessed the gusto to start the program. In addition, having been a former quick-fix, fad-diet devotee, she did not want her family and friends to see her trying to lose weight again and ultimately not succeed.

I assured Cara that the weight loss approach she was about to embark on was different and would ensure her long-term success. I also encouraged her to pick a "buddy"—it could be me or her husband or a close friend—to discuss her weight loss ventures with. However, I stressed that her venture was personal and it was her decision to share or not share with others. Instead of announcing to the world her new approach and her intention to get control and lose the weight (which is something I do not recommend), it was best for Cara to venture on this journey with one to two staunch supporters by her side. Cara realized that there would always be something that could prevent her from getting started and that she just needed to take charge here and now.

GETTING RID OF YOUR LIMITATIONS

Everyone has a "something"—a roadblock that needs to be cleared in order to be able to embrace change. Whatever life stage you are in at this moment, taking control and changing your diet, losing the weight and feeling like the energetic "you" you were meant to be will spill over so positively in every area of your life, you'll look back and wonder why you didn't do it sooner. I could fill pages and pages writing about the dramatic life transformations I have been witness to as I watched people first take control of their diets and lifestyle—people who worked night shifts or travelled a lot, people who were going through a divorce or who had just lost a loved one, and those who gained weight simply because life got busy and took over. The point is, the changes these people implemented made them feel better and made them far better equipped to deal with life's ups and downs. Although it may sound odd, I have seen several individuals finally land the job they want, become more peaceful with their children and spouse and be more active participants in life once they lose their excess weight. These people are not better because they have lost weight (they were lovable before and they will be lovable after!); they simply feel and look better, which causes them to do better. As highly acclaimed motivational speaker Jim Rohn once said, "You can't do well if you don't feel well."

Of course, as I mentioned, we are more than what we eat, but what we eat can propel us to new heights in every area. The right time to start is always now.

ARE YOU AN EMOTIONAL EATER?

There is a big difference between emotional hunger and physical hunger. Consider this scenario. Your boss calls to say he needs that report on his desk two days earlier than your original deadline. At the same time, your child is sick with the flu and you've been up all night playing nurse. Before you even realize it, your hand is in the cookie box and you have consumed three cookies to soothe your stress, nervousness and anger. How did that happen? Without any conscious awareness, food became your crutch and the friend you turned to when you were feeling upset.

If you can relate to this scenario, you are not alone. On some level we all have the capacity for emotional eating and use food or alcohol to soothe or "numb out" to a certain degree. Of course, there will be those times of extreme stress when we follow the "$%@# it!" rule—when we throw all caution out the window and eat or drink whatever we like—but the real issue arises when these faulty eating patterns become instilled as long-term behavioural strategies to deal with stress.

I have studied the habits of my weight loss clients for years and have probed the what, when and why behind their eating patterns. What I have discovered is that there are certain higher-risk times of day when we tend to eat for emotional reasons rather than because we are hungry.

Typically, emotional eating (or drinking) occurs:

- at 3 p.m.—to boost energy and ward off stress
- after dinner—cravings heighten and sweet binges occur to try to improve your mood and get a temporary boost
- when you are alone at night—a reward for a hard, stressful day

Rarely do I encounter a client who starts her emotional eating at breakfast. In fact, most people start their day off quite healthy and in control, only to crash and burn near the end of a long day. To determine if you are eating because of stress or for emotional reasons, see if you say yes to any of the following questions:

- Do you experience intense cravings for sweets?
- Do you tend to reward yourself with a drink or a snack late at night?
- Do you find food occupies your thoughts a lot of the time?
- Do you experience food guilt after you overeat?
- Does your dietary intake determine your mood?
- Do you sometimes put food in your mouth without realizing it?
- Do you prefer to eat alone?
- Do you eat in front of the TV or computer screen or in a parked car?
- Do you find yourself opening the kitchen cupboards or fridge if you are stressed, anxious or worried?
- Do you weigh yourself more than once per day?

If you answered yes to two or more of these questions, part of your relationship with food may be related to your emotional state. Once you start eating because of your emotions, you upset your hormonal and blood sugar balance, reaching for sugary treats, the wrong type of carbohydrates or alcohol. (Sadly, we do not typically binge on vegetables during times of stress!) This creates more energy fluctuations, more cravings and more irritability. In addition, you start to gain weight, which only aggravates the situation. This is why, to hit it out of the park for long-term weight loss success, you must deal with both elements: the emotional and the physical hunger. As you will discover, part of putting an end to emotional eating is discovering your *why.* This step is critical because when you identify your triggers, you will be able to snap back into a state of conscious eating and awareness.

The Emotional Eating Cycle

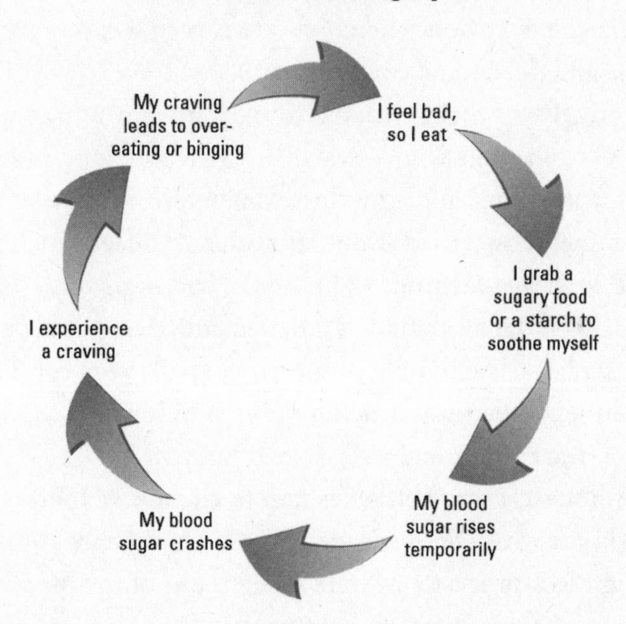

HOW TO FIND YOUR *WHY*

The point of this book is to teach you the nutritional tools you can use to lose weight permanently so that you will never again struggle with your weight. As I've said, for the results you are about to experience to become permanent, it is important to take the time to figure out your *why*. Again, while this may sound a little *out there*, I assure you there is nothing fluffy about this technique. The most successful companies and people in the world, from Apple and Nike to Oprah, all discovered their *why* before obtaining their results.

What I quickly realized in my weight loss practice was that the clients who pinpointed their *why* as the first step of their weight loss process were the ones who had breakthrough results. Remember, *weight gain is rarely about the food itself.* Some lifestyle habit, some stressor, some family history has trickled into your food behaviour and created a situation where you are carrying excess weight, feel lethargic and need to take back control.

Recently, I had a client name John. John was a highly successful 37-year-old man who worked in the technology industry. He arrived at my clinic for a first assessment with his wife, who was also extremely concerned about his health. At 6 feet 1 inch tall, John weighed in at an alarming 320 pounds, had high cholesterol, type 2 diabetes, snored at night, felt fatigued and, to top it off, smoked a pack of cigarettes per day. My inner alarm bells went off. This sweet young father of two was a ticking time bomb who was at extreme risk for a heart attack and a shortened lifespan.

To be honest, I was a little hesitant to encourage John to start off by figuring out his *why.* I was nervous he would balk at this part of the weight loss process and walk straight out of my office. Even so, I persisted and presented the *why* questions to him. To my surprise and delight, I couldn't have been more wrong. After some gentle probing, John's *why* answer spilled out of his mouth.

As a former athlete, John had known what it felt like to be fit, thin and energetic. Unfortunately, he had become extremely stressed out at work and had let his exercise regime and healthy eating habits fall by the wayside. He began to eat fast food 4 to 5 times per week and was drinking 3 to 4 cups of coffee per day to keep his energy high. Recent blood work revealed that his cholesterol and blood sugar levels were significantly elevated, and he was recommended a multitude of medications. John reported feeling out of control and slightly panicked. With an intense desire to get back on track, he was ready to take his first step back to health.

When I asked John why this was the right time for him to start a program, his answer was immediate, clear and concise: he had to lose the weight for his two children and his wife. He currently felt so fatigued and out of breath from his excess weight that he could not even carry his small children up the stairs. He also admitted that he was embarrassed by the way he looked and wanted to make his wife (who was quite well kept and attractive) proud of him. John's *why* was crystal clear. He would do whatever it took to get his health back for one good reason: his family.

John's honesty began a process that would dramatically change his health. By identifying his *why* he was able to clearly articulate that he had gained the weight because of the stress at work (situational) and the lack of time he devoted to himself. He also knew he wanted to lose the weight in order to be with his family for many more healthy and happy years. After John pinpointed his *why,* we continued on with the nitty-gritty part of his program, which I call the *do*—determining his metabolic ID, coming up with a plan to shift and balance his hormones and implementing the metabolic-boosting principles that would take him to the finish line—his goal weight.

In short, the three simple strategies for weight loss outlined in this book are:

1. Find your *why*—pinpoint why you gained the weight and why you want to lose it. This is your platform for success.
2. Do the *do*—after determining your metabolic ID, follow the personalized program to balance your hormones and blood sugars and

implement a plan to boost your metabolism and lose unwanted fat.

3. Enjoy your results—once you're here, you have "got it" for life. You have changed your set-up point, boosted your metabolism and are at your goal weight. A healthy weight, improved energy, improved mood, lower blood pressure and cholesterol, and stabilized blood sugars are all yours. No matter what situation, what stressor or life event is thrown your way, you will be able to deal with it without falling off the wagon.

Another example of a client who had enormous success by finding her *why* is Alexandra. Alexandra was a soft-spoken 30-year-old who came to my clinic the day after she and her boyfriend broke up. Feeling sad and beat-up confidence-wise, Alexandra still had the strength and wherewithal to show up for her initial appointment. Through her tears, she described feeling 10 out of 10 stress on a daily basis and giving in to her stress by emotional eating at the wrong time of day. At 5 feet 5 1/2 inches, she weighed 194 pounds and had a waist circumference of 40 inches. A highly regarded behaviour therapist, Alexandra was determined to get back to a weight that would make her feel good again and bring back her inner shine. Instead of focusing on the 50 pounds she wanted to lose (which would have been overwhelming for her anyway), we focused on *why* she wanted to lose it.

Alexandra clicked into the program and never looked back. Part of the reason she had gained the weight was the trouble caused by her relationship. Now, she had a strong *why* to lose it: to gain back a part of her life that was out of control, experience more energy and feel more like the young 30-year-old she was. The program prompted her to pinpoint the *why* and gave her the *do* part—that is, the tools for losing the weight, boosting her metabolism and creating a permanent lifestyle change. I am thrilled to tell you that Alexandra has lost 50 pounds and has a waist circumference of 31 inches (see before and after photos below). She has reached the final gratifying stage where she enjoys the results and maintains her new body. Overall she has lost 23 inches and looks and feels incredible. On her last day at the clinic when saying goodbye, Alexandra cried, but this time it was for a very happy reason. Seeing her incredible energy and new-found sense of confidence literally took my breath away.

What Alexandra says . . .

I was looking for change not just with my weight but with my life. I feel empowered now to take charge of my life because I have been given the tools to do so. I not only learned about nutrition and how to take care of myself but I learned how to live again and enjoy life. I realize now that my trepidation around losing weight was only because I thought I needed to sacrifice in order to gain what I wanted. I now see that I'm not sacrificing the things I love; rather, I can still enjoy the foods I love but just in a different way. The "side effects" of losing weight and getting healthy have been great! I now have an overall positive attitude and mood, glowing skin and shiny hair, and the aches and pains I used to complain about have completely vanished. Today I have more confidence to do the things I've always wanted to do but thought I couldn't. THANK YOU!

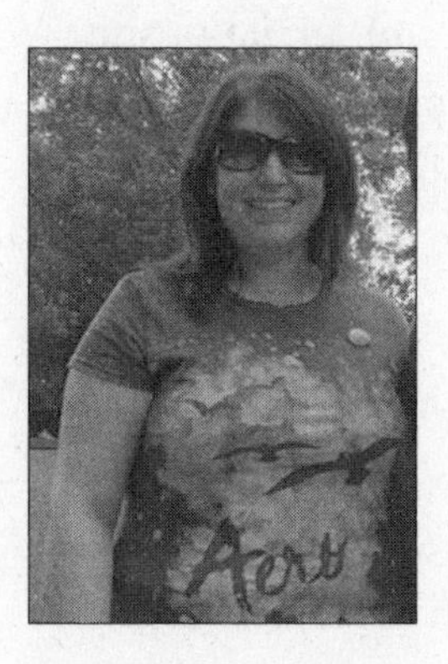

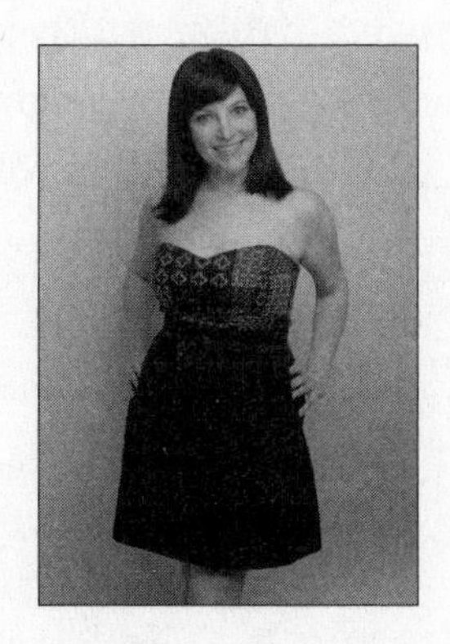

Alex lost
50 pounds

Are you ready to determine your *why?* All you have to do is take 10 minutes and ask yourself the two following questions, writing down your answers in the space provided. The answers are uniquely yours and do not need to be shared with anyone. But they are a fundamental part of your success—and they'll be fantastic to look back on as reminders once you have hit your goal.

1. Why did I gain the weight?

This is an integral question: you must identify and remove your emotional eating triggers before starting the program. If your job is enormously stressful and causes you to be sedentary and overeat, that is a critical thing to identify. Although this may seem like an obvious question, many people actually don't take the time to discover the underlying issue that started their faulty relationship with food. By thinking back to why your weight started to creep up, you will discover little "aha" moments that will help you to effect lifelong change.

2. Why do I want to lose the weight?

____

____

____

This second question will be the springboard to hitting your goal weight. Wanting to see your cholesterol drop, fit into your clothes comfortably, have more patience with your children or feel more like the energetic old you are all good reasons; identify yours and refer to them often along this journey, no matter how long or short it is.

I assure you: together, your answers to these two questions will begin the steps of building a health plan that works for you. Other potentially eye-opening questions that will help you stay focused on your *why* and be inspired to implement the *do* until you reach your goal weight include:

- How do I feel now?
- How do I want to feel?
- What is one thing I will do when I lose the weight that I am not doing now?

VISUALIZE: WHAT WILL I LOOK LIKE? WHAT WILL I FEEL LIKE?

After completing university, I followed in my sister's footsteps and went to school for chiropractic care. After graduating as a doctor of chiropractic, I opened what became a successful chiropractic clinic in Ontario. But I quickly realized I had a problem. Although I enjoyed seeing all of my chiropractic patients, my heart longed to practice nutrition full time. I truly believed I could have the greatest impact on people's health by teaching them the fundamentals of food and the impact it has on health and wellness. While I had (and continue to have) great admiration for chiropractors, I felt the practice was not my calling. This situation created quite a conundrum for me. I had just sunk thousands of dollars into a chiropractic practice and had spent even more on my schooling. I also had staff to pay, patients to take care of and commitments to honour. What to do? I felt stuck and even slightly depressed.

Instead of going into a deeper depression or panic mode, I took a very small first step. I began to visualize myself as a very successful nutritionist and writer. Whether during a walk, in the shower or while cooking, I would visualize a clear image of what my books and clinical practice would look like, and tried to tap into how I would feel having achieved these goals. At the same time, I started affirming with positive statements the goal I wanted to achieve—for example, "I am a very successful nutritionist." Over and over again, I would say these statements to myself to imprint what I wanted to occur.

Now, I do not attribute my successful career shift to visualizations and affirmations alone; however, they did start a momentum of change that spilled over into every area of my life. After I started visualizing, I implemented the *do* part by going back to school to become a registered nutritionist and started writing and publishing as many articles as I could. Lo and behold, 6 months after starting this process, I found the perfect chiropractor to buy my practice and the transition began. *The intention + the action = success!*

In addition to writing down your *why,* visualizing is an incredibly powerful exercise that will help you achieve your goal weight. Visualization has been shown time and time again to be a very influential tool for achieving your desires, with weight loss being no exception. We have all heard elite athletes describe how they saw in their heads the golf ball sinking into the hole, the baseball being hit out of the park or the puck shooting into the net. Wayne Gretzky describes how he continually visualized his hockey stick hitting the puck into the net time and time again. The act of visualization was part of his technique and training, and it helped him achieve his deserved title of The Great One.

The practice of visualization is gaining more and more acceptance in the medical world. Although mainstream science does not totally understand how visualization works, the fact of the matter is, it does work. The most interesting part of visualization is that it is effective even for those who are skeptical. I understand the skepticism—how can thought affect reality? The truth is, no one really has the answer. Whether visualizing creates a deeper neural pathway or whether there is something deeper going on, I assure you, the results from studies are clear: what you visualize will be more likely to occur than what you don't visualize.

To visualize weight loss effectively, you need to maintain a clear picture in your mind's eye of how you want your body, including your face, to look, while also tapping into how you want to feel. I tell my clients to follow the "fake it until you make it" approach. In other words, as you visualize, pretend that you already look and feel the way you want to be. This step will set your unconscious mind in motion to help you meet your weight loss goals. The clearer the images and the more you can tap into the feeling of how you want to be, the better. Thus, if looking at an old photograph of yourself or a picture in a magazine that resonates with you helps, go for it. When you are visualizing for weight loss, take 5 relaxed minutes of uninterrupted time to picture what you want to look like and try to imagine how looking that way will make you feel. Try to connect to the emotion, the feeling, the sense of the picture you conjure up in your mind. Connecting to the emotion will instill an even deeper relationship to the goal you are about to achieve. I also recommend using affirmative phrases, either silently or out loud, such as these ones:

- I weigh _________ (desired weight).
- I am energetic.
- I am healthy.
- I am in control of my food choices.
- I am strong.

Your affirmations will be far more powerful if they are in the present tense: "I am" versus "I will." And remember, affirmations are positive: "I feel energetic" rather than "I am not tired." Your subconscious will always respond better to what you stand for rather than what you are against. Again, it does not really matter at this point if you believe in visualization or affirmations or not. Once you start the practice, the proof will be in the results—inches down, pounds gone.

Of course, visualization alone will not take you to your goal weight, balance your blood sugars or break your cravings. You must incorporate the *do* part—the action steps outlined in the Metabolism Boosting Diet. However, as you have now discovered, to ensure your weight loss results are permanent you must deal with health and weight loss on two levels: the physical and the emotional. By dealing with both elements, you will achieve lifelong success.

PINPOINT YOUR PATTERN

In my practice I have a number of clients who have gained 10 or so pounds simply by having an evening snack each and every night. Tired after a long day and looking for a little pick-me-up, they were eating a bowl of cereal at night or a few cookies before going to bed. No big deal, right? Wrong! This evening snack may appear innocent and not really that high in calories, but it soon leads to bloating and blood sugar fluctuations, and it imprints a very bad pattern of nighttime eating.

Because losing weight is about more than just the food you are eating (or not eating), it is prudent to examine your behavioural relationship with food. Along with finding your *why* and visualizing your future success, a very effective strategy for ensuring a permanent shift is to identify your eating patterns. In other words, start to pay attention to the specific time of day or type of situation where you tend to fall off the health wagon and are triggered to eat or binge. For some, it may be excess alcohol on the weekends that keeps their weight high; for others, regular nighttime eating after dinner may be the root cause of their problem. It does not matter if you have 10 or 100 pounds to lose—everyone has a pattern. The first step before change is awareness. The more conscious you are of what and how you eat, the more likely it is that your results will be permanent. To help identify *your* patterns, fill in the blanks in the following statements:

- My healthiest meal is at _______________ (what time of day?).
- I tend to fall off the health wagon when _______________ (e.g., time of day, stressful situations).
- My go-to cheat foods include _______________.
- If I could just stop doing _______________, I think I could lose weight.

Remember, it is very hard to binge eat or eat unconsciously when you are paying close attention to your patterns.

WHAT DO I NEED TO START THE *DO* PART OF THE METABOLISM BOOSTING DIET?

Once you have removed your roadblocks and any perceived limitations and identified your *why*, you are ready to start the *do* part. Keep focusing on your reasons and your inspiration to take the weight off.

Whether it's to be able to run faster with your kids, improve your love life, feel and look younger, or decrease your menopausal symptoms, all reasons are the right reasons. Give yourself a pat on the back for taking the noble venture toward a healthier you. You are about to discover a whole new approach to eating and living that will thrill you. To start, all you need is a few simple tools and tips.

A GOAL WEIGHT

I ask my clients, "If I could wave a magic wand and make you any weight you would like to be, what would that weight be?" Most people instantly come up with the weight at which they felt their best. When determining your goal weight, be realistic. If you have never been 120 pounds, do not plan to hit that as a goal weight. And don't refer to height and weight charts for your supposedly ideal weight. Those charts, first developed for insurance company purposes, are mostly outdated. Your goal weight is the weight at which you felt like your most fit and energetic self. Identify it; you will later record it on your Metabolism Boosting Tracking Chart (more on that later). This will be the target you hit at the end of this process.

A SCALE

When it comes to buying a scale, I recommend a digital one, as needle scales have a greater margin of error. The scale does not have to cost hundreds of dollars. It simply has to take an accurate morning reading. If you purchase a scale that also measures body fat percentage, be aware that certain factors can affect that percentage, such as the amount of water in your body, your food intake, body temperature and recent physical activity.

Whichever scale you choose, I encourage you *not* to weigh yourself daily. By doing so, you may see fluctuations that are caused by the time of month, or a high-sodium meal that you ate the night before, or digestive issues (e.g., a short bout of constipation). If you become obsessed with the scale, you risk letting your emotions get the better of you. All you need to do is take your morning weight once or twice per week (pick a day or two that will be your weigh-in day) and record it on your Metabolism Boosting Tracking Chart (see page 272). Since you may weigh up to 2 to 4 pounds (1 to 2 kg) more in the evening, it is of the utmost importance that you weigh yourself at the same time of day, for consistency, and wear the same type of clothing. Women should also keep in mind that they may weigh more before and during the menstrual cycle.

A MEASURING TAPE

You'll need a measuring tape to take three measurements each week: waist, hip and chest circumferences. A cloth or plasticized sewing tape measure works best. You'll find instructions on how to take the measurements on page 43.

I am a big advocate of keeping pictures of yourself before you begin your weight loss journey, perhaps holding on to a pair of pants (that will soon be huge on you!). As you'll discover once you're in the MAINTENANCE phase, these photos will be a testament to just how significant your health changes are.

THE METABOLISM BOOSTING FOOD JOURNAL

Research shows that those who keep a food journal will lose more weight in the long run compared with those who don't. Remember, you are far less likely to binge eat or eat off-plan when you're mindful and recording your food and beverage intake. On page 271 you will find a sample food journal. Use yours for a minimum of 1 month (longer is always recommended).

THE METABOLISM BOOSTING TRACKING CHART

This chart, found on page 272, will be your weekly monitoring system for weigh-ins. Record your weekly or biweekly weight and inch loss on this chart. This will be a quick and easy way to track your results. The measurements I recommend taking per week are waist, hip and chest circumferences. Those keeners who love to track their success with lots of numbers can also measure their thigh and bicep circumferences.

The Metabolism Boosting Tracking Chart works. The reason? Once you see your results and continue measuring your success, you will be motivated to continue. Let's face it: weight loss has a domino effect—the better you do, the better you will want to do.

A BUDDY

Everyone needs a "buddy" or someone to be accountable to when losing weight. When I was losing weight after having my baby, my buddy was my sister. To be accountable and have a check-in system, I e-mailed her every night a description of what I had eaten that day. Simply knowing I had to report to someone at the end of each day encouraged me to continue with my weight loss. If you do not wish to share your weight loss journey with anyone, that's not a problem—your buddy will be your food journal.

A DECLUTTERING SESSION

Although not a tool per se, the decluttering session is an important initial part of the program. After the first few days, when you are balancing your hormones and blood sugars, you will find that your cravings subside and you don't "need" sugary treats or starchy foods as much. You may indulge in them once in a while, but the uncontrollable desire for them (which is not a sign that you are weak but rather that you are hormonally and biochemically "off") will be gone. However, before beginning the program, it is important to declutter your kitchen to remove all of your temptations—candy, chips, cookies or whatever they may be. You will eventually be able to have these foods in your home; however, in the first few days, you may find that your cravings *increase.* At the height of a craving, it is very difficult to make the right food choice, and those goodies that put on the weight in the first place will likely win out. So get rid of them!

TAKING YOUR MEASUREMENTS

Below I outline a number of ways for you to measure your weight loss success. Remember, the more numbers you have to show progress, the better. After all, who doesn't like to see good results?

MEASURING YOUR WAIST, HIP AND CHEST CIRCUMFERENCES

Measuring waist circumference

1. Remove any clothing and accessories so that you can measure your waist on bare skin.
2. Stand with your feet together.
3. Starting at the top of one hip bone, bring the tape measure all the way around your waist, level with your navel.
4. Making sure that the measuring tape is not too taut, relax and exhale (i.e., do not hold your breath), then take the measurement.

Healthy waist circumferences for most adults:

Men: Less than 40 inches (102 cm)
Women: Less than 35 inches (88 cm)

For people of South Asian descent, a healthy waist circumference differs slightly:

Men: Less than 35 inches (88 cm)
Women: Less than 32 inches (80 cm)

Measuring hip circumference

1. Stand with your feet together.
2. Placing the measuring tape around the widest part of your buttocks, take the measurement.

Measuring chest circumference

1. Stand with your feet together.
2. Bring the tape measure all the way around your torso, level with the broadest part of your chest.
3. Making sure that the measuring tape is not too taut, relax and exhale (i.e., do not hold your breath), then take the measurement.

BODY MASS INDEX

Body mass index is a calculation that uses your height and weight to estimate how much body fat you have. The equation is:

BMI = body weight in kilograms divided by height expressed in metres squared.

Body mass index (BMI) categories

- Underweight < 18.5
- Normal 18.5 to 24.9
- Overweight 25.0 to 29.9
- Obese ≥ 30.0

Risk of Associated Disease According to BMI and Waist Size

BMI	Weight Category	Waist 40 inches (102 cm) or less for men or 35 inches (88 cm) or less for women	Waist 40 inches (102 cm) or greater for men or 35 inches (88 cm) or greater for women
< 18.5	Underweight	N/A	N/A
18.5 to 24.9	Normal	N/A	N/A
25.0 to 29.9	Overweight	Increased	High
30.0 to 34.9	Obese	High	Very high
35.0 to 39.9	Obese	Very high	Very high
≥ 40.0	Extremely obese	Extremely high	Extremely high

Source: http://www.consumer.gov/weightloss/bmi.htm

BODY FAT PERCENTAGE

Pounds can lie, body fat percentage cannot. In other words, two people can be of the same height and weight but have two very different amounts of body fat.

Body fat percentage is simply the percentage of your weight that is made up of fat. The part that is not fat is referred to as lean body mass. For example, a 160-pound man with a lean body mass of 130 pounds has 19% body fat. This may sound high but it's not, when you consider that a certain amount of fat is necessary to insulate the body and protect internal organs.

A few key points to keep in mind when it comes to body fat percentage:

- Women have more body fat than men. This is partially due to fatty breast tissue and increased fat accumulation around the hips. If her fat levels drop too low, a woman may stop menstruating.
- Men have more total muscle than women and therefore have a lower body fat percentage.

- As people age, their total muscle mass decreases and fat increases.
- Body fat percentage and body mass index (BMI) are two separate calculations that should not be confused. BMI is a calculation based on height and weight, not body fat percentage.

How can I determine my body fat percentage?

There are several methods to determine your body fat percentage, and they vary in accuracy. Unfortunately, the more accurate the method, the more hassle and the more expensive it tends to be. The options from most accurate to least are as follows:

- ***DEXA scan***—a full-body X-ray using bone density. Very accurate.
- ***Hydrostatic weighing***—weighing done while completely submerged under water. Very accurate.
- ***BIA (bioelectrical impedance analysis)***—scales and/or hand-held devices run a low level of electrical current through the body; the resistance between the conductors provide the body fat measurement. Although such testing tends to be fairly accurate, and is the method I tend to use in my practice, results can vary according to time of day, the client's level of activity that day and hydration. Try to have the BIA test done in the morning after drinking a glass of water. Do not take this test if you have a pacemaker or if you are pregnant.
- ***Skinfold caliper testing***—a very simple test that estimates body fat percentage by measuring skinfold thickness. Measurements can be taken on three to nine anatomical sites. However, there is often wide variation in the results, depending on who conducts the test.
- ***Navy tape measurement***—a formula based on measurements taken with a tape measure. I find it rather confusing to explain to clients and often not very accurate.

Age-Adjusted Body Fat Percentage Recommendations

Women

Age	Underweight (%)	Healthy (%)	Overweight (%)	Obese (%)
20–40	< 21	21–33	33–39	> 39
41–60	< 23	23–35	35–40	> 40
61–79	< 24	24–36	36–42	> 42

Men

Age	Underweight (%)	Healthy (%)	Overweight (%)	Obese (%)
20–40	< 8	8–19	19–25	> 25
41–60	< 11	11–22	22–27	> 27
61–79	< 13	13–25	25–30	> 30

Source: D. Gallagher et al., "Healthy percentage body fat ranges: an approach for developing guidelines based on body mass index," *American Journal of Clinical Nutrition*, 2000, 72(3):694–701.

Once you have gathered all the necessary tools, you will be on the road to success, just like my client Darlene. A 64-year-old nurse practitioner who stands 5 feet 3 inches tall, Darlene first arrived at my clinic weighing just over 231 pounds, with a BMI of 40.9. Darlene had been diagnosed with type 2 diabetes and was having trouble controlling her blood sugars. She also had sleep apnea, a condition where a person stops breathing for short periods during sleep, which forced her to use a CPAP machine at night (a CPAP machine has a mask that fits over the mouth and nose, or just over the nose, and gently blows air into the throat). Married and working full time, Darlene had an extremely busy life filled with travel, young grandchildren and business meetings. By the time she arrived at my clinic, she had experienced her weight loss "aha moment," when she knew she would have to make a change to keep up the pace of life she wanted. Darlene was about to take the plunge to discover her new self.

I am happy to report that as I write, Darlene has lost 63 pounds and 10 inches from around her waist. She is even down one full shoe size. Once a size 22, Darlene now fits into a size 12. Happy, energetic and able to shop for brand new clothes, she has a new lease on life and looks and feels fantastic. Congratulations, Darlene!

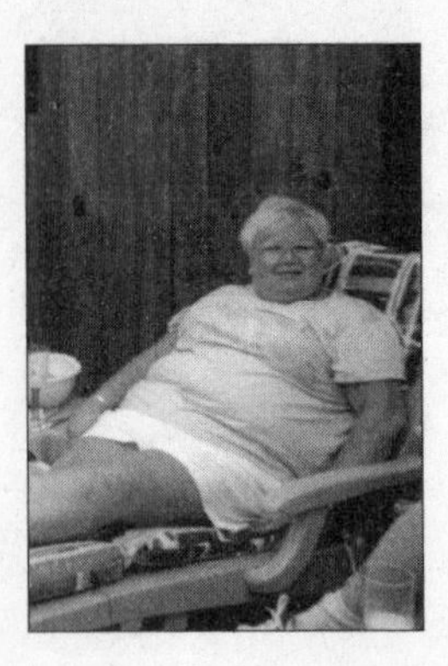

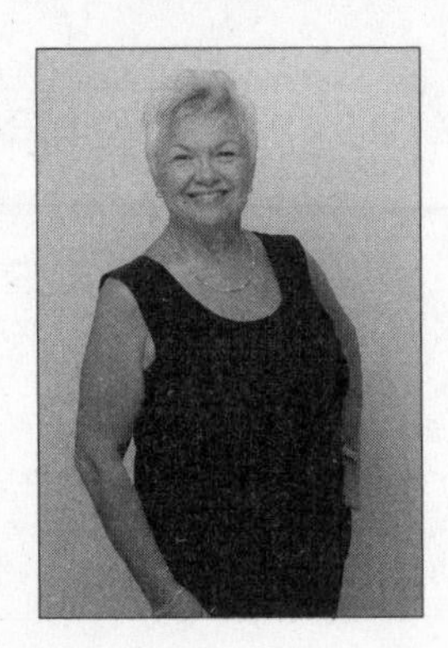

Darlene lost 67 pounds!

CHAPTER 3
MEET YOUR METABOLISM

He that takes medicine and neglects diet wastes the skill of the physician. —Chinese proverb

I'd like to reintroduce you to someone: your metabolism. Whatever age or stage you are at in your life, you are about to "make friends" with your metabolism and learn how to change your set point and boost your personal metabolic engine for maximum fat loss. By understanding how to rev your metabolic engine with the principles outlined in this book, you will develop a lifelong tool for keeping your weight off. You may be eager to begin the program immediately and skip to Chapter 6 to take the Metabolic ID Questionnaire. However, I encourage you to take the time to read this chapter and the next two, as they provide the foundation for a successful start and will build the platform for long-term success.

WHAT IS METABOLISM?

Simply put, metabolism is the chemical process that converts the food we eat into fuel for the body. As soon as you take a bite of a sandwich or a sip of orange juice, your metabolism clicks on like the engine

> Metabolism is the amount of energy (calories) your body burns to maintain itself. Whether you are eating, drinking, sleeping or exercising, your body is constantly burning calories to keep you going.

of a car. Similar to the gas that runs the car, our food and beverages are the sources of fuel that run the body. Several factors determine the life of a car and how smoothly it runs—the quality of fuel we use, the regularity of tune-ups and oil changes, weather conditions and so on. Similarly, our body's metabolic engine has influencing factors that can help or hinder our weight loss efforts. The key is to drive your metabolism in the proper direction without overtaxing it. Pushing your metabolism to the extreme over and over again (as with fad or crash dieting) will eventually cause your metabolic engine to fail.

Just as everybody has a unique metabolism, everyone has a unique basal metabolic rate (BMR). Your BMR is defined as the number of calories your body burns at rest: in other words, how many calories your body burns simply by running its everyday functions like breathing, sleeping and digesting. Some people have a slow metabolism and others have a very fast one, but we all possess a considerable degree of flexion or wiggle room. In this book, I frequently use the term *set point* in referring to one's metabolic potential. A set point is the regulatory system that maintains the body at a certain weight. The set point can be likened to a thermostat for body fat. Let's say, for example, there is an outside temperature of 30 degrees Celsius and you would like your air conditioner to maintain an indoor temperature of 23 degrees. No problem—your AC will not have to work too hard to cool your home by 7 degrees. However, if outside temperatures soar to 40 degrees, your AC will not be able to cool your home as efficiently and will struggle to keep the indoor temperature at 23 degrees. Almost undoubtedly, the indoor temperature will be warmer than the 23 degrees programmed. Why? The gap has become too big.

This is precisely what happens with your set point. If over a long period, outside variables change (e.g., you eat too many processed foods, or you are significantly stressed or sedentary), your set point will adjust upward and you will gain weight.

> The metabolic set point is an internal survival mechanism to ensure there is adequate body fat in the event that food becomes scarce. Unfortunately, in modern times, our bodies no longer distinguish between a famine and a crash diet and so tend to store excess weight and fat if the dietary approach is overly restrictive.

Many people think their set point is stuck and their metabolism cannot ever be boosted. These are typically the same people who go on extreme caloric-reduction diets. But as you will soon discover, caloric intake is only one piece of the puzzle. In truth, everyone's metabolism has the capacity to change. The key is to properly set off your metabolic alarm in order to reset your set point.

FACTORS THAT CAN ALTER YOUR METABOLIC RATE

Numerous factors can influence the efficiency of your metabolism and the rate at which you burn fat. The Metabolic ID Questionnaire in Chapter 6 takes into account all of these factors to determine a personalized weight loss program that is most suitable for you. Even if you identify with one, two, three or more of the influencing factors outlined in the next few pages, you *can* and *will* change your

> The United States has the highest obesity rate in the world and also the highest number of people on diets.

metabolism's potential. Through my years of practice, I have not "met" a metabolism that I couldn't budge. Although some metabolic engines at first need a bit more "sparking" than others to balance out chronic hormonal imbalances or a history of yo-yo dieting, to date I have found that, if you follow the program, it works each and every time.

Read on to learn about the factors that can alter your metabolism's potential and rate of burning fat. Most of these factors can be balanced or altered to put the proper pressure on your metabolic engine, change your set point and effect change.

STRESS

Mild to moderate stress reactions can trigger cortisol response. Cortisol is a stress hormone secreted by your adrenal cortex that may promote the excess storage of fat. The intensity and the length of stress are often influencing factors in cortisol activity. Thus, experiencing mild to moderate short periods of stress (e.g., I've lost my wallet!) does not tend to elevate cortisol levels as much as prolonged periods of intense stress (e.g., a family illness, a divorce, a crisis at work). In addition to causing weight gain, elevated cortisol levels can wreak havoc on blood sugar levels, blood pressure and overall immune system function. The good news is that proper dietary and lifestyle practices can very quickly and easily normalize elevated cortisol levels.

EATING TOO MANY HIGH-GLYCEMIC-INDEX CARBOHYDRATES AND STARCHY FOODS

High-glycemic-index foods, explained in more detail on page 64, tend to trigger the oversecretion of the hormone insulin. As you will soon learn, excess insulin equals excess fat storage. In a nutshell, the glycemic index (GI) is a measure of the speed of entry of a carbohydrate into the bloodstream. The faster the entry, the higher the secretion of insulin and the more fat storage, cravings and hunger you'll experience. Examples of high-GI and no-no starchy foods are white breads, cookies, cakes, muffins, certain cereals, instant oatmeal, pretzels and instant mashed potatoes.

Combine high-GI foods and emotional eating and you get weight gain. This is why I am not an advocate of programs that merely count calories. In essence, you can count the wrong calories, which can make your weight loss slow and frustrating and, furthermore, will not put you in a state of optimal health. Counting calories long term also breaks my rule about whether you see yourself following the program in 5 years' time. If you cannot see yourself counting calories or points for the rest of your life, does such a diet really make sense?

EATING TOO LITTLE FAT

I cannot tell you how many times I encounter someone trying to lose weight who is stuck in the old low-fat way of thinking. Wanting to lose weight, he or she dodges fat intake at every corner. But when it comes to weight loss, your body must have enough of the good type of fat to lose weight—the fats found in nuts, seeds, avocados, certain oils and fish. Without proper fat intake on a daily basis, your metabolism will "think" it is starving and cling on to your body fat. In fact, recent research demonstrates that adding more "good" fat into the diet in the form of omega-3 essential and monounsaturated fats actually helps to lower overall body mass index. You may be surprised to learn just how much good fat you can eat on the Metabolism Boosting Diet and still lose weight. More on that later.

HORMONAL IMBALANCES

Numerous hormonal imbalances—from peri-menopause and menopause to thyroid dysfunction, hysterectomy, fibroids and polycystic ovarian syndrome—can cause a disturbance in the proper functioning of your metabolism. The most common hormonal imbalance for a woman is when she hits menopause and experiences a drop in estrogen; for a man it's when he hits andropause and experiences a drop in testosterone. These stages of life are inevitable. Many people report finding it harder to lose weight at this time of life and soon discover fat deposition in undesirable locations, including the abdominal region.

While weight loss is different at this life stage, it certainly can be achieved with the proper metabolic tools. I frequently witness the positive weight loss results of people 55 and older once they discover the Metabolism Boosting Diet (in fact, one of my dearest weight loss clients is an 83-year-old woman). Fat deposition does not have to occur in the abdominal region or contribute to the love handles or apple body shape that is a risk factor for various diseases, including cancer, heart disease and stroke.

INACTIVITY

The body needs a combination of anaerobic (brief and intense) and aerobic (longer lasting, less intense) activities to keep the metabolism running at high speed, prevent bone loss, improve cardiovascular health and build muscle. That said, you do not have to hit a gym for an hour of intense physical activity every day. The Metabolism Boosting Diet workout suggestions detailed in Chapter 7 involve shorter workout times at higher intensities. They are fast and easy and can be done in the privacy of your home.

POOR SLEEP

If you do not get enough sleep, your neuroendocrine control of appetite (the brain's feedback loop on appetite) can become upset, leading to insulin resistance, storage of fat around the abdomen and eventually type 2 diabetes. Lack of sleep also affects your body's ability to regulate leptin, a hormone that tells you when you have received enough food and to stop eating. Inability to fall asleep, frequent waking up and light sleeping can all contribute to excess weight.

After the age of 30, your body gradually begins to lose muscle. If your activity level and the amount of calories you eat stay the same, you will gain weight because your metabolism has slowed down. You must rev up your metabolism in a very specific way to boost your engine's potential.

As well, the risk of sleep apnea is higher for people who are overweight. A person with sleep apnea may suffer from daytime sleepiness, difficulty focusing and even cardiac disturbances. The excess fat stored around the neck can make the airway smaller, causing difficulty breathing. The good news is that losing the weight and regular exercise can often have dramatic positive effects on sleep apnea.

DEHYDRATION

To lose weight and ensure proper functioning of the digestive system, your body has to be well hydrated. Unfortunately, North Americans are prone to being dehydrated, typically opting for coffee, sugary pops, flavoured water (loaded with sugar), diet drinks and juice as their beverages of choice—all drinks that are dehydrating diuretics. For hair and skin health, digestion, energy and total well-being, I recommend following the Metabolism Boosting Diet's steps for sneaking more water into your food and beverages on a daily basis (more on this later).

FAULTY DIGESTION

Faulty digestion and an inability to lose weight often go hand in hand. On a first visit to my clinic, it is not uncommon for a client to report being constipated, feeling bloated or suffering from irritable bowel syndrome. Why does this occur? Simply put, the foods and dietary patterns that add the weight in the first place are the same foods and dietary patterns that contribute to the clogging and inflammation of the digestive tract. If you've read any of my previous books or attended one of my seminars, you'll recognize this statement: "You are only as healthy as your pipes." In other words, you need to absorb and digest your food properly (and have a minimum of one bowel movement per day) for weight loss to occur. This is why my weight loss approach has a heavy emphasis on proper digestion. That way, not only will you benefit from proper daily elimination, but without the bloating, you'll have a flatter stomach.

REACTIONS TO MEDICATION

Certain medications, including antidepressants, can have a slowing effect on the metabolism. I'm not suggesting you go off your medication. However, there are dietary and lifestyle changes you can make that will compensate for unwanted weight gain from meds.

FOLLOWING A VERY LOW-CALORIE DIET (VLCD)

Severe caloric restriction, which is often touted by crash diets, has been shown to be ineffective for long-term weight loss success. In fact, a severe drop in calories can have the exact opposite effect on metabolism, slowing your metabolic engine and encouraging more fat storage in the long run. In addition, very low-calorie diets (frequently referred to as VLCDs) often result in binge-like behaviour and encourage an unhealthy relationship with food.

BEING A CHRONIC YO-YO DIETER

The one thing the body hates more than carrying excess weight is chronically gaining and losing it. If you are a lifer in the weight loss world, you are doing a number on your metabolism and it is time to stop. It is not uncommon for my clients who have been on countless diets—high-protein, calorie-restricted, "food by mail," meal-skipping, shakes-only and so on—to report not being able to lose even 1 pound in a week. As you will see, to correct the problem, you need to first identify your metabolic ID, begin to change your set point, shift to a balanced state and then implement the steps that will boost your metabolism.

EMOTIONAL EATING AND FOOD BINGES

At my clinic, we offer evening seminars on a variety of topics. The seminar series that always attracts a full house is the one on emotional eating. Let's be honest: if weight loss were about "just the food," few people would have a weight issue. But we all have some emotional connection and relationship with food, faulty or not. However, getting balanced and boosted on the Metabolism Boosting Diet will eliminate your cravings and nighttime eating patterns. Happy, bored, sad, lonely or stressed—whatever your feelings, you need to make peace with food.

Pinpointing your *why,* as described in Chapter 2, also helps put an end to emotional eating. As I said earlier, emotional eating episodes tend to occur in the evening hours or when you are alone. Unfortunately, mindless eating tends to clog up your digestive pipes and upset the blood sugar balance that your metabolism thrives on. Thus, it slows down your "engine," leaving you feeling bloated, stuffed and beaten down. I assure you, you can and will change this cycle. Let your motto be "Lose the weight, live my life." Very soon you will be able to eat with enjoyment and without guilt.

CHRONIC NIGHTTIME EATING

Many of my clients report that their eating habits are "perfect" until after dinnertime. In other words, they start their day off healthy by eating a great breakfast but find themselves finishing their day off with too many sugars, a few too many calories and some mindless eating and/or drinking. Nighttime eating typically has an emotional basis (you feel sad, bored, lonely, stressed, unplugged) and is not cued by true hunger. I cannot tell you how many teachers I have had as clients who gained weight over the years by stress-eating in front of their computers during report card season. Stressed out and working late nights to complete the reports, these hard-working teachers start to overindulge in "reward" foods. Without even realizing it, they begin to tip their blood sugars, start to crave more sugars and starches and incorporate all the wrong behaviours for weight loss and energy boosting.

What I tell these clients and other nighttime eaters is that the timing of your eating does impact your ability to lose weight. According to Ayurvedic medicine (an ancient Indian form of medicine extolled for its holistic and healing properties and popularized by Dr. Deepak Chopra), your digestive and metabolic capacity is strongest in the early afternoon (from 1 to 3 p.m.), making lunch the most important meal of the day. As the sun goes down, so does the potential of your metabolism. Thus, making dinner your largest meal and noshing after dinner on cereal, cookies, candy or chips will slowly but surely pack on excess weight and make digestion and elimination sluggish.

Now that you understand how your metabolism works and its influencing factors, let's move on to Chapter 4 to discover how matching and mixing certain macronutrients can help with weight loss, blood sugar balancing and boosting metabolism.

CHAPTER 4

FOOD AND THE PLAYERS ON YOUR TEAM

Happiness lies, first of all, in health.
—George William Curtis

For best results on the Metabolism Boosting Diet, it is helpful to have a working knowledge of the players on your team. By understanding the basic mechanisms of how macronutrients are utilized by the body and how they influence your hormones and control blood sugars, you can in turn utilize them in a specific manner to lose fat, build muscle and stay at your goal weight.

MEET THE TEAM: THE MACRONUTRIENTS

Macronutrients are the "big guys" that your body requires daily to run efficiently. There are three categories of macronutrients: carbohydrates, proteins and fats. When choosing macronutrients, the key is to focus on the types that must be included in your diet, rather than on the types that should be eliminated. Although I'll identify the no-no foods that trigger excess weight gain, hormonal imbalances and a sluggish metabolism, my main goal here is to open you up to a world of food choices that are so delicious and nutritious, you won't feel as if you're missing out on anything. As a dedicated foodie, I truly believe that food is one of the great pleasures of life, and that it should be enjoyed and relished on a daily basis.

There has been a lot of confusion around dieting and the macronutrients. In the 1980s, carbohydrates were all the rage. People were consuming mass quantities of pasta, breads and potatoes in order to lose weight. In the 1990s, carbohydrates were out. Enter fats. Low-fat foods were the big thing, and avoiding fat to lose weight was the key to a slimmer waistline.

By 2000 and onward, protein was—and still tends to be—king. Eating protein to lose weight and feel fit was (and still is) a popular campaign. Following high-protein diets (for example, an Atkins approach) allows people to drop weight very fast, but this weight loss is not sustainable long term if the other two macronutrients, carbohydrates and fats, are not properly integrated into the diet. As you will see, in addition to proteins, proper proportions of carbohydrates and fats must be consumed for long-term weight loss success.

If we were to step back for just a moment and really look at the patterns, it is obvious that the magic-bullet approach to weight loss persists and merely jumps from trend to trend. Although there is some merit to each of the approaches mentioned above, on their own they do not offer balance or a long-term strategy that can be sustained for life.

Luckily, the science that is now available in the field of integrative health care (once called alternative health care) has grown by leaps and bounds. The research on what types of the macronutrients are needed for weight loss is now abundantly clear. As you will discover in later chapters, the key to success is variety: eat various amounts and types of the three macronutrients in order to balance blood sugars, boost metabolism, balance hormones and lose weight. By eating in the manner outlined in the following pages, you will have numerous options to choose from, all of which will take you to your goal weight for life.

All the foods in the Metabolism Boosting Diet contain at least one of the following attributes:

- anti-inflammatory
- low on the glycemic index
- high in antioxidant value (see Appendix 1, page 273, for a list of such foods)
- nutrient-dense, calorie-light
- rich in fibre
- energy-boosting
- hydrating

In terms of weight loss, people run into trouble with macronutrients on two fronts. First, they drastically reduce or completely eliminate one of the macronutrients from their diet (for example, they opt for a no-fat diet or eliminate carbohydrates altogether). But any diet that drastically reduces or eliminates one of the three macronutrients is not a diet that is based on long-term healthy eating behaviour and therefore typically has temporary results. Keep in mind the question "Can I see myself following a version of this program in 5 years' time?" If you can't, don't do it. The cycle of gaining–losing–gaining back more is even worse than never losing the weight at all.

The second mistake people make is selecting poor-quality macronutrients (refined flours and sugars, saturated fats, products filled with additives or preservatives, etc.). This approach typically results in heightened cravings or hunger and increases the risk for numerous diseases and health conditions, including high cholesterol, acid reflux, joint pain, irritability, depression, inflammation and digestive issues. This is why diet programs that merely count calories and do not focus on food quality do not propel you toward optimal health and wellness. A diet filled with low-fat products (which often contain aspartame, sucralose and food dyes) or filled with empty calories (refined, floury goods or high-fat food such as cakes, cookies, candy, chips, only in smaller portions) often results in food binging and a sense of being on a strict diet. If you feel like you are fighting it out with your diet, chances are you'll end up losing the battle.

So, now that we understand that each macronutrient on the team plays an important role in weight loss and the overall maintenance of optimal health, it's time to meet the players.

PLAYER #1: CARBOHYDRATES—THE FUEL PROVIDERS

Carbohydrates are found in fruits, vegetables, grains and legumes, among other foods, and are the main source of fuel for your system. Your body breaks down carbohydrates into glucose, which is the sugar that the runs the entire show for your brain and the rest of your body. Without carbohydrates, the body must seek out fuel from other sources, including fat, which is not nearly as efficient a fuel. For weight loss success and thriving health, your system must be fed a constant supply of high-quality fuel, and this will come from the proper intake of carbohydrates.

In years past, the mantra of many weight loss seekers was "Cut carbohydrates." I have had far too many clients cut out a majority of all carbohydrates—even nutritious grapes, bananas and carrots—in an attempt to shed excess weight. These clients end up feeling fatigued and even dizzy from lack of fuel in their diet.

On the Metabolism Boosting Diet, the emphasis is on eating the right type of carbohydrates, those that do not make blood sugars fluctuate, increase cravings, upset hormonal balance or cause weight gain in the abdominal region. These types of carbohydrates are classified as low-insulin secretors and are also low on the glycemic index (more on this later; also, you'll find a listing of foods and their glycemic index value in Appendix 3). Ideally, your carbohydrates should be derived from fruits, vegetables and a modest amount of whole grains and legumes every day. The amount of carbohydrates you eat per day will vary according to the phase of your program. Once you determine your metabolic ID (see Chapter 6), you will know precisely how much to consume daily.

When it comes to carbohydrates, many weight loss seekers have grown accustomed to hearing about the glycemic index. All foods are given a value on the glycemic index (GI) according to the extent to which they raise blood sugar levels after being consumed. The categories are as follows:

- Low-GI food: < 55
- Medium-GI food: from 55 to 70
- High-GI food: > 70

The process of high-GI carbohydrate digestion and its potential weight-gain cycle works like this:

1. You eat a food that is high on the glycemic index, such as a cookie, muffin or pretzel.
2. Your blood sugars rise quite rapidly.
3. The rapid rise in blood sugars triggers your pancreas to secrete the hormone insulin, which lowers blood sugars by allowing for the uptake of sugar from the bloodstream into your cells.

4. When you overconsume foods that rate high on the glycemic index and you are also inactive or overweight, your body tends to oversecrete the hormone insulin. In other words, your body tends to become unresponsive to your insulin.
5. Your pancreas responds by secreting more and more insulin. When this occurs, your blood sugars will drop too low.
6. Low blood sugar, called hypoglycemia, will result in fatigue, mental fuzziness and cravings for more sweets and high-GI carbohydrates. We often refer to this as the 3 p.m. slump or having a sweet tooth, rather than linking it to the quality of carbs we've just eaten.
7. To compensate for the symptoms of hypoglycemia, our body sends our brain a message—what we call a craving. Unfortunately, we tend to crave simple sugars (found in specialty coffees, cookies, crackers, candy) to bring blood sugars back up and start the vicious cycle of overeating the wrong types of carbohydrates all over again.
8. The excess insulin that was secreted triggers the storage of excess glucose. But instead of being stored as glycogen in the liver and muscles as is normal, the excess is converted to fat and stored around the midsection (abdominals). The cycle of eating high-GI foods and giving in to the resultant cravings soon triggers excess weight and, depending on your genetics, can lead to type 2 diabetes, heart disease, high cholesterol or cancer.

Take a look at the graphs on page 67. The first one illustrates the dramatic fluctuations in blood sugar levels that result from eating high-GI foods. There is a constant, large up-and-down swing in sugars. This triggers a variety of unwanted symptoms (sluggish metabolism, fatigue, mental fuzziness) and eventually can lead to heart disease, cancer, high cholesterol and type 2 diabetes. The key is not to eliminate one macronutrient completely; rather, it is to choose the proper types and proportions of macronutrients to maintain balance. As you can see in the second graph, which illustrates blood sugar fluctuations once on the Metabolism Boosting Diet, you will still have these fluctuations, but the spikes will be far less intense. By getting into balance, you will experience sustained energy throughout the day, improvement in mood, far greater weight loss and, best of all, no more cravings.

YOUR BRAIN NEEDS GLUCOSE TOO!

Neurons (brain cells) cannot utilize alternative energy sources like fatty acids to any significant extent and therefore rely on glucose, the sugar derived from carbohydrates, to feed the brain. Lack of glucose in the diet can make you feel dizzy, fatigued and foggy.

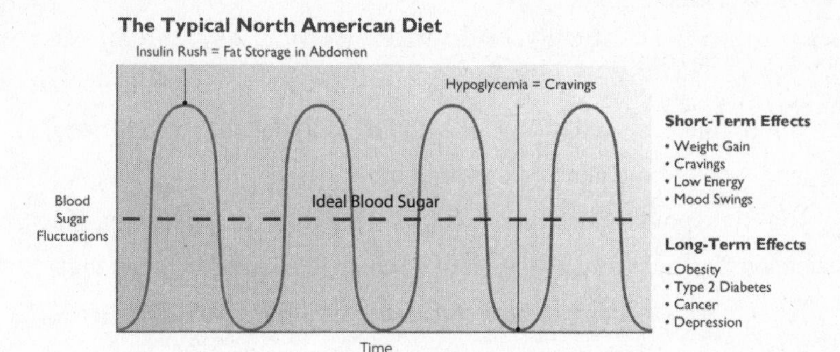

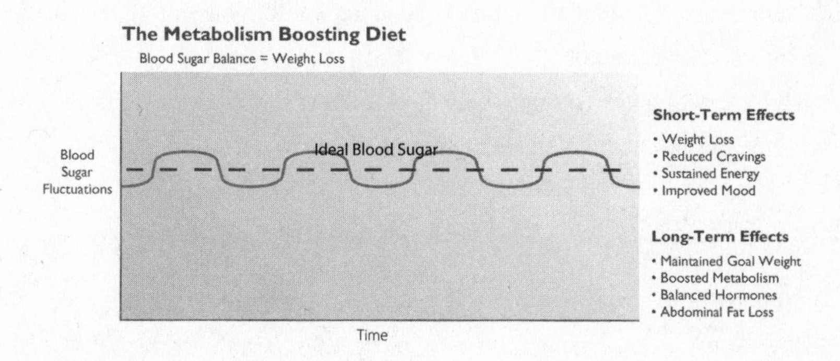

Although the glycemic index gives us a very good idea of the body's insulin response to certain foods, it has its limitations. One of them is that it does not identify other characteristics of the foods, such as calories, antioxidant capacity, anti-inflammatory properties and nutrient density, or lack thereof. For example, peanut M&M's are not an ideal choice for weight loss, but they do have a GI rating that is low at 41. This is because fat, protein and fibre all act as brakes, slowing the entry of carbohydrates into the bloodstream. Thus, the fat-filled peanut in an M&M lowers its GI rating. What this rating does not tell you is that this food is high in inflammatory fats, high in calories, contains food dyes and can easily trigger more cravings because of its added sugars.

Other limitations of the glycemic index are:

- The GI rating is significantly affected by food ripeness, processing, length of storage and cooking method.
- The GI response can vary markedly from person to person depending on insulin sensitivity. Some foods have an insulin index rating that reflects the insulin response they generate. These results are preliminary and further research needs to be done.
- Most of the values on the GI do not show the impact of glucose after two hours. Yet some diabetics have blood fluctuations for up to four hours after eating.
- A food with a low GI rating may have a high carbohydrate content (e.g., certain pastas) and vice versa.

> On the Metabolism Boosting Diet, you will be getting approximately 35% of your calories from high-quality, low-GI carbohydrates during the weight loss phase and approximately 40% of your calories from carbohydrates during the MAINTENANCE phase.

WHAT'S THE DIFFERENCE BETWEEN GI AND GL?

GLYCEMIC INDEX

The glycemic index, or GI, was developed in the 1980s by Dr. David Jenkins at the University of Toronto. The original goal of the GI was to help people better manage their diabetes. Since then, the GI has been shown to have significant uses for proper weight management.

To measure the GI of a carbohydrate, a serving providing 50 grams of available carbohydrate is given to 8 to 10 participants. Their blood sugar levels are then measured over a period of 2 hours. The subjects' response to the carbohydrate being tested is compared to their response to 50 grams of pure glucose. The first response is divided by the second and multiplied by 100. The average blood sugar response will determine the GI value of that food.

GLYCEMIC LOAD

The glycemic load (GL) takes the serving size (i.e., the number of grams of carbohydrates) into account. The GL is calculated by multiplying the GI by the amount of available carbohydrate in a serving divided by 100. The term "available carbohydrates" refers to the amount of digestible carbohydrates (i.e., the amount of carbohydrates left after subtracting dietary fibre from the total). The GL rankings are as follows:

0 to 10 = low
11 to 19 = medium
20 and up = high

See Appendix 3 for a detailed listing of the glycemic index value and the glycemic load of various foods.

The Metabolism Boosting Diet meal plans and recipes take into account the glycemic load (GL) and the glycemic index (GI) response. As you will see, keeping blood sugars in check and eating carbohydrates that do not overstimulate insulin production is indeed part of the equation in the Metabolism Boosting Diet, but it is not the entire story.

For maximum weight loss results, your dietary intake on the Metabolism Boosting Diet will consist of carbohydrates from vegetables, certain fruits, and a modest amount of legumes, fibre, starches and grains depending on your plan. White sugars and white flours will not be part of the plan. In addition to ranking higher on the glycemic index, these types of foods tend to lower immune system response, zap energy and create an endless cycle of cravings that is not conducive to hitting your goal weight.

Refined sugars

White refined flours and white sugars are major contributors to the obesity epidemic our society is experiencing today. Of course, most foods that contain refined flours and white sugars rank quite high on the glycemic index and trigger the secretion of insulin. When you eat these foods, your body over time will become insensitive

DID YOU KNOW THAT STUDIES SHOW:

- Children who eat a high-GI breakfast continue to consume 53% more calories before suppertime than children who eat a low-GI breakfast.
- Infants born to women with high-GI food consumption patterns have higher body fat than those born to women who typically eat lower-GI foods.

to its own insulin and start to secrete more and more in an effort to open up the "doors" of the cells.

Take, for example, my client Tanya. Tanya first came to see me weighing 207 pounds. Given her height of 5 feet 8 inches, that weight put her body mass index of 31.5 in the obese category (see Chapter 2 for more details on body mass index). Although Tanya was extremely active, doing boot camp classes on a regular basis and walking her dogs each morning, she could not lose a pound. At the young age of 39, with two kids to raise and a busy job, she was fed up, tired and ready for a change.

When I reviewed Tanya's diet, it was obvious that she had a serious sweet tooth. She told me that it typically reared its ugly head at 3 p.m. when her energy dipped or at night while she was working on the computer. Tanya had an admitted "chocolate problem" and was also treating herself to

THE LOCK AND KEY FUNCTION OF INSULIN

The effect of insulin has been compared with that of a lock and key. In each cell is a "door" that can allow glucose (sugar derived from carbohydrates) to enter. However, this door stays locked until insulin comes around with the "key" to open it. When insulin is present and the "door" is "unlocked," glucose can enter the cell and be used as fuel for the body. As glucose leaves the blood to enter the cell, the amount of glucose remaining in the blood is reduced. In this way, one of the main roles of insulin is to lower blood glucose. If blood glucose is lowered too much, however, a state of hypoglycemia (low blood sugar) can result, inducing feelings of fatigue, mental fogginess and cravings for sweets.

cookies, ice cream, bagels and pizza when she felt stressed or rushed. She acknowledged often eating because of intense cravings and stress rather than true hunger. While on paper it looked like Tanya was doing most things right (working out, drinking eight glasses of water per day), it was obvious why she was stuck.

I assured Tanya that she was not alone and definitely not weak; however, she was biochemically unbalanced from her food choices. I also told her if she tried to fight her cravings, it would not work. After determining Tanya's metabolic ID, I started her on the first step of the Metabolism Boosting Diet. I knew she had to get her blood sugars regulated (recall those mini peaks illustrated in the second graph on page 67, versus the major peaks in the first graph) in order to break her cravings and begin the weight loss process.

Tanya clicked into the program beautifully and hasn't looked back. She is one of my weight loss superstars, losing from 3 to 5 pounds per week. She now weighs in at 160 pounds and has a normal body mass index of 24.3. She is well aware that white sugar is a major no-no for her and can easily trigger cravings and weight gain. Although Tanya still has stress in her life thanks to her demanding job, she has made a focused effort not to turn to white sugar for comfort. When she is tempted to fall back into her old ways, she reminds herself of the sugar hangover and knows it is just not worth it. Tanya turns to other sweet substitutions (small amounts of dark chocolate, frozen fruits and certain supplements) to keep herself satisfied.

Tanya lost
47 pounds

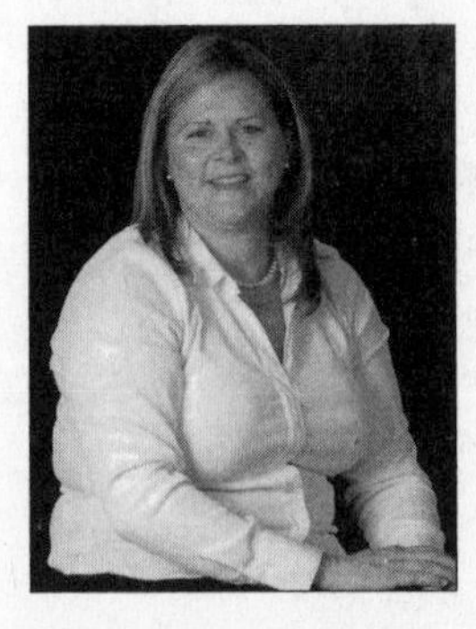

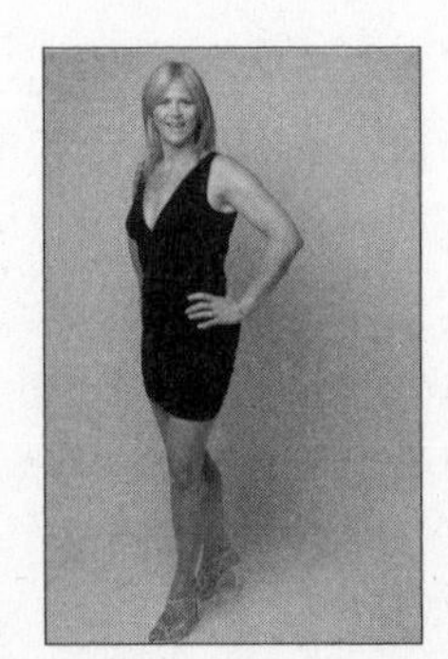

Where does white sugar hide?

White sugar is snuck into many foods these days. In addition to causing weight gain, energy fluctuations and intense cravings, white sugar can also suppress immune system function and lower white blood cell count. It was always interesting to me that the children in my chiropractic and nutritional practice used to come down with a cough or cold the first week in November. It finally occurred to me that many little ones were getting sick after binging on sugary Halloween candies! The white sugar was contributing to the crash in their immune system and allowing viruses or bacteria to which they were exposed to take hold.

To become sugar savvy and minimize the amount of refined sugars in your diet, simply follow these suggestions:

- When picking a cereal, choose one that has less than 7 grams of sugar per serving. Since 4 grams of sugar equals 1 teaspoon (5 mL), if you are eating a cereal with 16 grams of sugar per serving, you are eating 4 teaspoons (20 mL) of added sugar.
- When reading a label, if the first few words end with "ose" (e.g., glucose, sucrose, galactose, maltose, dextrose, fructose), the product contains a lot of sugar. Other names that sugar goes by are honey, corn syrup, maple syrup and juice concentrate.
- Do not be scared of fruit. Fruit does not contain added sugar. Part III details optimal weight loss fruits on the Metabolism Boosting Diet.
- Do not switch from sugars to aspartame to save on calories. Research indicates that in addition to being potentially toxic, aspartame can actually increase hunger and cravings over the long run. It is not uncommon for me to meet with someone at my clinic who has 40 or more pounds to lose but also drinks four or five diet sodas per day. Don't do it!

- Be aware of foods that contain an abundant amount of sugar, such as ketchup, sports drinks, fruit-bottom yogurts, juices (especially cranberry juice) and certain morning bars or cereals.

WHAT IS HIGH-FRUCTOSE CORN SYRUP?

High-fructose corn syrup is a cheap sweetener that is often added to juices, sodas and other processed foods. The sweetener has become enormously popular with certain manufacturers, as it appears to extend a food's shelf life. However, research has clearly indicated that the body does not treat this substance the same way as other sweeteners and that it promotes weight gain and fat deposition around the abdomen. A recent study at the University of California had one group eat high volumes of high-fructose corn syrup and another group eat high volumes of regular white sugar. After 10 weeks, the former group had new fat cells surrounding their vital organs, while the latter group had no additional fat cells. In short, this sweetener is a big no-no on the Metabolism Boosting Diet. When reading labels, beware: high-fructose corn syrup may be cleverly disguised as corn sugar.

PLAYER #2: PROTEIN—THE STABILIZER

The second member of the macronutrient team is protein—the stabilizer—so called because it lowers insulin response, stabilizes blood sugars, cuts cravings and creates a feeling of satiation. Protein triggers the release of a hormone called glucagon, which breaks down fat. In essence, insulin and glucagon have opposing effects. Insulin stores fat, glucagon breaks it down. However, both hormones are equally vital to the good functioning of your body. You cannot run your body on straight protein to lose weight; it must have carbohydrates as the primary source of fuel to sustain life.

Protein is composed of "building blocks" called amino acids. There are 20 amino acids in total. Eleven are non-essential, meaning our body can make them, while the remaining 9 are essential and must be supplied by our diet. Animal proteins (fish, chicken, beef, eggs and most dairy products) and soy proteins used to be called complete proteins, since they contain all 9 essential amino acids. Plant proteins also contain all essential amino acids, but they can be low in one or more of them (these are referred to as "limiting amino acids"). Proteins are no longer classified as complete and incomplete. Combining proteins is unnecessary because by eating a variety of plant foods the body breaks down the protein into individual amino acids, which contributes to a "reserve" in the amino acid pool. As long as we eat proteins regularly throughout the day, our cells tap into this pool.

OPTIMAL PROTEIN OPTIONS

- chicken and turkey
- fish: salmon, tuna, haddock, halibut, cod, sea bass, snapper, herring, mackerel, sardines, swordfish
- shellfish: crab, lobster
- cottage cheese
- yogurt
- eggs and/or egg whites
- whey protein isolate powder
- red meat in moderate amounts (choose the round cut, top sirloin, shank, round flank or chuck for red meat lower in saturated fat)
- tempeh, tofu, soy (for more information, see pages 279–81)
- legumes: edamame, chickpeas, black beans, etc. (can also be used as a vegetarian option)

Protein is one of the integral macronutrients needed for losing weight effectively. You will find that when you begin the Metabolism Boosting Diet, the weight you lose is not from muscle wasting; rather, it is from pure fat loss and typically comes off the abdominal and hip region first. You will be able to accurately monitor your inch loss week by week by using the Metabolism Boosting Tracking Chart found on page 272. The quality lean protein choices that are recommended as part of the diet will also help to improve fitness, immunity and antioxidant function and to enhance and regulate insulin and leptin release (leptin is a hormone that makes you feel full).

Proper protein intake for weight loss is an integral part of the Metabolism Boosting Diet because it does the following:

- boosts metabolism
- cuts cravings
- creates feelings of satiation
- helps to maintain muscle mass, which is important for fat loss
- helps to balance and stabilize insulin

The amount of protein required for good health depends on many factors, namely body weight, age, physical activity, state of health and environment. As a general guide, the RDA (recommended dietary allowance) for protein is 0.8 grams per kilogram of body weight for adults.

Daily Recommended Intakes of Protein

Age	Protein (grams/day)
Infants	
0–6 months	9.1
7–12 months	13.5

Children	
1–3 years	13
4–8 years	19
Males	
9–13 years	34
14–18 years	52
19–30 years	56
31–50 years	56
51–70 years	56
> 70 years	56
Females	
9–13 years	34
14–18 years	46
19–30 years	46
31–50 years	46
51–70 years	46
> 70 years	46

Source: Food and Nutrition Board, Institute of Medicine "Proteins and amino acids." *Dietary Reference Intakes for Energy, Carbohydrates, Fiber, Fat, Fatty Acids, Cholestero,l Protein, and Amino Acids (Macronutrients)*, 2002/2005, www.nap.edu.

I find that the RDA recommendations for protein given in the preceding chart tend to be on the low side for effective weight loss results and that, for ultimate weight loss results, protein intake has to be significantly higher (approximately 60 to 80 grams for women per day and 80 to 100 grams for men per day). In fact, several studies have shown that increasing levels of protein helps those wanting to lose weight by increasing the loss of body fat and reducing the loss of muscle tissue. During the initial weight loss phase of the Metabolism Boosting Diet, you will be getting approximately 30% to 35% of your calories from lean proteins.

PLAYER #3: FAT—THE CONDUCTOR

Fat is the third macronutrient and the big "conductor"—it provides the pathways for nerve conduction that are necessary for every cell in your body to communicate with each other. Fats are also vital to hormone production, proper vitamin utilization, maintaining healthy blood flow in the arterial walls and the building of healthy brains. As powerful anti-aging agents, fats are a must-have and can do wonders for the skin (clearing up acne, reducing signs of aging) and hair.

When it comes to weight loss and fats, the research is in and is abundantly clear: *the right types of fat are integral for hormonal balance, boosting metabolism and ultimately weight loss results.* You will be surprised at just how much "good" fat you can eat on the Metabolism Boosting Diet and still lose weight. I always remind my clients that, as a general rule, fat does not make you fat. The obesity epidemic we are experiencing has several causes, including the consumption of too many refined flours, a high-stress lifestyle, lack of sleep or activity and hormonal fluctuations. Rarely do I have a client who is overweight from overconsuming butter! This is not to say that you can get all of your calories from fat and lose weight, but the right type of fat is actually your friend when it comes to boosting your metabolism effectively.

There are several types of "good" and "bad" fat. The fats to be aware of are these:

Monounsaturated fats (MUFAs)

Monounsaturated fats, or MUFAs, well known for their heart-healthy properties, have long been a staple in the Mediterranean diet. Examples of MUFA sources are nuts (walnuts, almonds, peanuts, pistachios, macadamias, hazelnuts), oils (olive, peanut, canola), seeds (pumpkin, sesame, sunflower) and avocados. MUFAs are an integral part of the Metabolism Boosting Diet, as research has shown these types of fat to be necessary for proper weight loss and achieving a healthy body mass index (BMI).

Olive oil is one of the most studied monounsaturated fats and is the superstar of the MUFA world because of its health benefits. Extra-virgin olive oil (made from the first pressing of the olive) has been shown to do the following:

- lower LDL (the "bad cholesterol") levels;
- reduce the risk of a cardiovascular incident (like a heart attack);
- offer a rich source of vitamin E, a powerful antioxidant;
- offer a rich source of plant nutrients called phytonutrients, which provide protection against a variety of diseases, including cancer and heart disease.

Olive oil is suitable for cooking on medium heat. It can also be drizzled over vegetables or brown rice, added at the end of cooking to a stir-fry, or used to make sauces and heart-healthy dips.

Fats suitable for cooking on high heat include ghee (clarified butter), butter, sesame oil, grapeseed oil and coconut oil. See Appendix 4 for a more detailed list of the healthiest fats to cook with.

Polyunsaturated fats (PUFAs)

When it comes to polyunsaturated fats, or PUFAs, it is important to make the distinction between the sources. There are certain PUFAs, such as our beloved omega-3s, that are incredibly valuable for overall health and weight loss. On the flip side, refined vegetable oils such as safflower, corn, sunflower and soybean, which also fall into the category of PUFAs, tend to be not so good for overall health and wellness. North Americans typically overconsume omega-6 polyunsaturated fats in the form of these refined vegetable oils, which drives down omega-3 essential fat levels and can lead to inflammation. And although PUFA vegetable oils have been shown to lower "bad" LDL cholesterol, they have also been shown to lower "good" HDL cholesterol when eaten in excess. As well, PUFA oils are very sensitive to heat, making them susceptible to rancidity. This is why they should be stored as they are usually sold, in dark bottles rather than clear ones.

The good PUFAs, the ones that should be maximized in the diet and are a must for weight loss, are the essential fatty acids (EFAs). These fatty acids are called *essential* because they cannot be made by the body and must be derived from the diet. They have several roles in the body that are critical to overall health and wellness. Vital jobs omega-3s are responsible for include the following:

- maintaining a healthy cell membrane to allow the intake of nutrients and the outflow of toxins
- maintaining flexibility in cell walls to ensure proper communication from cell to cell (specifically important for neuronal cells—a.k.a. brain cells)
- decreasing inflammatory response (e.g., arthritic pain, digestive complaints)
- offering cardiovascular protection
- improving cognitive function
- assisting with mild to moderate depression
- anti-aging effects, such as improving the look of skin and reduction in fine lines*

In terms of weight loss, several studies have demonstrated that

* For more information on how to improve the look and feel of your skin, see Appendix 1, pages 273–275, the Metabolism Boosting Diet's 7-step skin protocol.

essential fatty acids assist with feelings of satiety and help reduce total body mass index. For example, in 2007, the Landspitali University Hospital in Iceland conducted a study to determine the effect of fish or fish oil supplements in weight loss diets for young adults. At the end of the 8-week study, men had lost an average of 14 pounds and women an average of 9 pounds. The highest weight loss occurred in the group that consumed omega-3–rich fatty fish 3 times per week.

For our purposes, there are two basic types of essential fatty acids to be aware of:

1. **Omega-3 fatty acids**. Three particularly important types of omega-3 EFAs are critical for health and weight loss. The first, alpha-linoleic acid (ALA), is found in flaxseed, soybeans and canola oil. ALA is also found in small amounts in certain vegetables, including kale, spinach and Brussels sprouts. The second type is docosahexaenoic acid (DHA). This, along with eicosapentaenoic acid (EPA), the third type, is generally found in cold-water fatty fish (salmon, cod, mackerel, tuna) as well as in fresh seaweed. The body partially converts ALA to EPA and DHA; however, the conversion is not very efficient. This is why I am a big advocate of supplementing with a high-quality distilled fish oil.

2. **Omega-6 fatty acids** (linoleic acids or LAs). Linoleic acid is the main type of omega-6. It is found in abundance in soy oil, sunflower oil, safflower seeds and oil, sesame oil and corn oil. Due to overconsumption of refined vegetable oils found in processed foods, the typical North American diet contains far too much omega-6. The ideal ratio of omega-6 to omega-3 is 2:1. At the moment, the ratio is closer to 20:1. This ratio is believed to be a significant contributing factor to the development of chronic inflammation and other chronic diseases.

With the Metabolism Boosting Diet, a significant amount of EFAs is incorporated into the daily food plan, as they are very effective at reducing total fat mass and sustaining permanent weight loss results. Ideal omega-3 food sources are cold water fish, fish oils, flaxseed and flaxseed oil, omega-3–fortified foods, walnuts and walnut oil and soybeans. Optimal sources of omega-6 are raw nuts, seeds, borage oil, grapeseed oil and primrose oil.

Saturated fats

Saturated fats, found in meat products, butter, cheese, whole milk and ice cream, among other foods, are typically solid at room temperature. A small amount of saturated fats (approximately 5% to 7% of total caloric intake) is allowed on the Metabolism Boosting Diet and will not hinder your results.

One issue with saturated fats is that, when eaten in excess, they can create an inflammatory response in the body. Have you ever noticed that when you eat a meal rich in fried foods, cheeses or red meat, you feel bloated or puffy, or your joints feel achy the next day? This is because the food you consumed (likely in excess) is inflammatory and can exacerbate pre-existing conditions. In fact, one study, the results of which appeared in the *American Journal of Clinical Nutrition,* found that within an hour of eating a meal filled with saturated fats, participants experienced an increase in inflammatory proteins that are associated with heart disease. Levels of these inflammatory proteins remained elevated for three to four hours.

CALORIES IN THE THREE MACRONUTRIENTS

Carbohydrates = 4 calories per gram
Proteins = 4 calories per gram
Fats = 9 calories per gram

Another issue with saturated fats is that, when eaten in excess, they can raise "bad"

LDL cholesterol and can contribute to plaque buildup and the clogging of arteries. (More about cholesterol on page 84.)

Trans fatty acids (TFAs)

Trans fatty acids, or TFAs, first became popular when food manufacturers discovered TFAs could extend a product's shelf life. Instead of only three to six months, shelf life could be extended to years.

When a liquid vegetable oil is flooded with hydrogen at a very high temperature, trans fatty acids are formed. This process changes the shape of the fat into an unnatural one (from a semi-circular fat to a straight-chain fat). In other words, what was once a liquid is now a solid fat. Most TFAs are found in processed foods such as baked goods (muffins, cakes, cookies), crackers, snack foods and fried foods (donuts, french fries, onion rings). Along with being void of precious nutrients necessary for optimal health, foods with high TFA levels can raise the "bad" LDL cholesterol and lower the "good" HDL cholesterol. This can increase your risk for high blood pressure and cardiovascular incidents such as heart attack and stroke.

The best way to avoid TFAs is to take a moment to read the food labels. As of 2006, several countries, including Canada, have legislated that all packaged foods must list the presence of TFAs. The amount of trans fatty acids will be listed under the amount of saturated fat on the Nutrition Facts table. (You'll

> Eating fat has little effect on your insulin levels, and it actually decreases your appetite. Also, eating the right kind of fats can rebalance hormones and improve the way you look and feel.

find a sample Nutrition Facts table in Appendix 2.) Also look for the words *partially hydrogenated, hydrogenated* or *shortening* in the ingredient list, which indicates the presence of TFAs. The daily recommended amount of trans fatty acids on the Metabolism Boosting Diet is zero.

On the Metabolism Boosting Diet you will be consuming approximately 30% of your calories from fat sources. The good fats found in monounsaturated fats and omega-3 and omega-6 fats will be the mainstay of your fat sources.

THE CHOLESTEROL STORY

Cholesterol is a waxy substance that occurs naturally in the body. It is a type of fat called a lipid, which is vital in making cell membranes, vitamin D and hormones. In healthy people, about 80% of their cholesterol is produced by the body. The rest comes from what they eat.

Cholesterol can't dissolve in the blood. It has to be transported to and from the cells by carriers called lipoproteins. There are two types to be aware of:

1. **Low-density lipoprotein (LDL)**. Of all the forms of cholesterol in the blood, LDL cholesterol is considered the most important form in determining the risk of heart disease. Treatment decisions such as exercise, diet and medication are often based on LDL values. LDL carries cholesterol from the liver to the body cells. LDL cholesterol has been termed the "bad" cholesterol because, when there is too much of it, plaque can build-up in the arterial walls and the risk for heart disease increases significantly.

2. **High-density lipoprotein (HDL)**. Referred to as the "good" cholesterol, HDL cholesterol moves the opposite way of LDL. In other words, HDL particles return extra cholesterol to the liver for disposal.

HEALTH CANADA GUIDELINES FOR CHOLESTEROL

- Total cholesterol: less than 5.2 millimoles per litre (mmol/L) is ideal and more than 6.2 mmol/L is high.
- HDL cholesterol: more than 0.9 mmol/L is ideal.
- LDL cholesterol: less than 3.5 mmol/L is ideal and more than 4.0 mmol/L is high.

Next time you have blood work done, keep a copy of your levels. If your numbers are off, have them retested after you lose 15 or more pounds.

TO RECAP

- All three macronutrients—carbohydrates, protein and fat—are necessary in specific types and amounts to lose weight and balance hormones and blood sugars.
- Glucose, derived from carbohydrates, is the fuel that runs your body.
- Ideal carbohydrate choices are those that are nutrient-filled and low on the glycemic index.
- An oversecretion of insulin, a fat-storage hormone, can be triggered by eating too many of the wrong types of carbohydrates.
- Glucagon, a hormone triggered when protein is consumed, breaks down fat.
- Protein satiates and is a stabilizer of energy and blood sugars.
- Fat is necessary for weight loss.
- Ideal fats to cook with include olive oil, if using medium heat, and ghee (clarified butter), sesame or coconut oil, if using high heat.
- Fat, fibre and proteins act as brakes that slow the entry of glucose into the bloodstream (and therefore lower the insulin response).

- For maximum fat loss on the Metabolism Boosting Diet, you will primarily be eating a delicious diet filled with low-insulin-secreting foods, lean proteins and fats from the MUFA and EFA categories.

Once you get the hang of the Metabolism Boosting Diet, you will be making specific macronutrient choices to drive up your metabolic potential and change your set point to burn fat and balance hormones. Once you do this, cravings, lack of energy and the need to eat old comfort foods will be a thing of the past.

CHAPTER 5
THE TRIANGLE OF WEIGHT LOSS

Life is not merely to be alive, but to be well.
—Marcus Valerius Martialis

If you were to walk into my weight loss clinic, you'd see the big sign in the waiting room that reads "Shulman Weight Loss—simplify, simplify, simplify." The purpose of the sign is to instantly put my clients at ease and to assure them that the program will be straightforward, based on science and suitable for any and all lifestyles. I have found that, with all the clutter in the weight loss world—from diets emphasizing heavy-duty detoxes to those with a strict caloric mantra of "Calories in, calories out"—people are becoming confused and frustrated. With the pile of what-to-do-to-lose diets growing at a rapid pace, it is time to get back to the basics of what works and make it simple.

In order for you to maximize fat loss and enter a disease-prevention mode, the Metabolism Boosting Diet bases your dietary intake on three core elements:

1. Hormonal health
2. Quality calories
3. Optimal digestion

The Triangle of Weight Loss

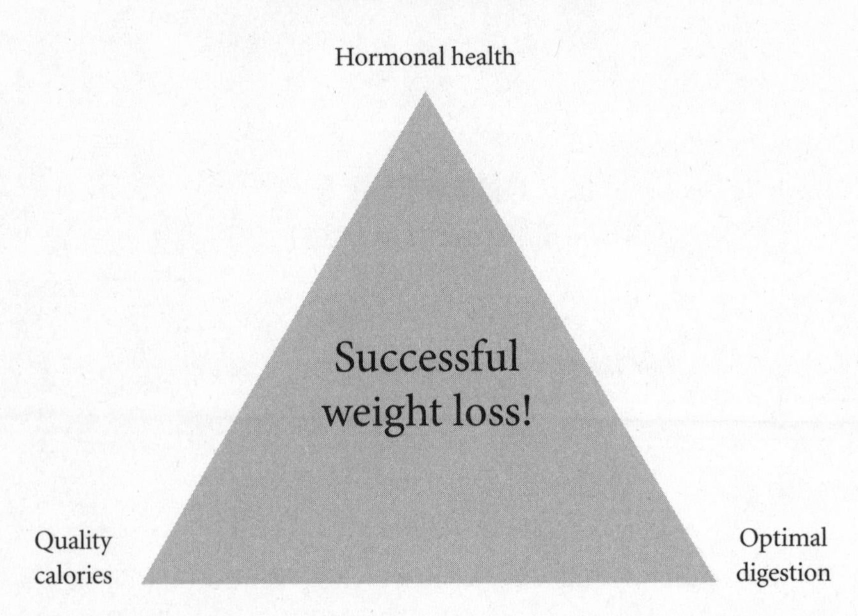

Do not panic—I promise not to bore you with a detailed scientific explanation of each of these three elements. Remember, the goal is to keep the process extremely simple so that you have principles in your "back pocket" for weight loss that can be applied at the office, at home, on vacation or during times of stress. That said, I will be providing you with just enough "need to know" information about all three elements. Once you have finished reading this book, you will be a knowledgeable student of nutrition, empowered with information that will serve you for a lifetime. Each of the three elements outlined in this chapter is integral for your weight loss success. When you put all three together in a delicious eating plan—presto! Results for life, and a tool you can return to in times of cheating and overindulging. Your friends will wonder why they continually gain and lose weight while you find your weight loss results effortless to maintain.

THE OPPOSING HORMONES

Insulin: a hormone that promotes fat storage

Glucagon: a hormone that breaks down and burns fat

CORE ELEMENT #1: HORMONAL HEALTH

Ah yes, your hormones. Hormones are the most powerful chemical messengers in the body, and when it comes to weight loss, they can make it or break it. In addition to blood sugar control and insulin balance, hormones control metabolism and therefore are intricately connected to the amount of fat you gain or lose. In other words, burning fat and achieving successful weight loss is in fact partly a hormonal event. The good news is that hormones are fluctuating and can change depending on a variety of factors, such as stress levels, stage of life, physical activity and dietary food intake.

The Metabolic ID Questionnaire I'll ask you to complete in the next chapter takes into account your hormonal history as one of the key influencers of overall body weight and metabolic functioning. Your answers to the questionnaire will determine the most effective program for you to help you hit your goal weight. As mentioned in Chapter 4, one of the primary focuses of the Metabolism Boosting Diet is to balance blood sugar, insulin and glucagon levels. Remember, an oversecretion of insulin triggers fat storage, especially around the abdominal section, whereas glucagon has an opposing role, breaking down fat. To change your body composition permanently, you must get the ratio of insulin to glucagon in check. This is why a "calories in, calories out" approach alone will not work—hormonal balance must be achieved.

Insulin and glucagon are key players when it comes to losing weight and burning fat, but they are not the only ones. Hormones are all interconnected—they can be likened to a very sophisticated and in-depth telephone network. In other words, all hormones "talk" to each other and can have effects in various areas, from body weight and digestive health to overall mood and sense of well-being. When it comes to diet and exercise, hormones can be dramatically influenced and balanced by specific food choices, supplements and lifestyle activities. In fact (and pay attention, this is a key point), hormones react differently to proteins, fats and carbohydrates and can support or impede weight loss. Since hormones are constantly "chatting" with each other, once one falls into place, so to speak, the others tend to respond as well. The table below lists those hormones in the body that are intimately involved in weight loss.

Hormones and Weight Loss

Hormone	Function	Imbalances	How to balance
Insulin	Secreted by the pancreas, it regulates glucose levels by lowering blood sugar. Promotes fat storage. Lowers blood sugar after a meal but in excess promotes fat storage and inhibits fat burning.	Excess secretion of insulin can trigger hypoglycemia (low blood sugar), excess fat storage and cravings.	Exercise, eat regularly to keep blood sugars stable, ensure sufficient protein and fat in the diet, reduce stress. Eat adequate fibre and fat and eliminate artificial sweeteners.

Hormone	Function	Imbalances	How to balance
Glucagon	Has the opposite function of insulin, increasing glucose levels. Breaks down fat. Released when blood sugars drop (from skipping a meal or restricting calories). Helps release stored fat for fuel.	A decrease in glucagon is related to an increase in insulin, which leads to fat storage in the abdominal area.	Increase lean protein options in the diet.
Cortisol	Secreted by the adrenal glands in times of stress or when insulin levels are high.	High levels can trigger fat storage and a drop in the hormone DHEA, which helps to build muscle. Increases appetite and cravings for sugar and simple carbohydrates, as well as belly fat.	Meditation, exercise, a balanced diet and various supplements can all be very helpful.
Testosterone	Important in both males and females, it regulates metabolism, maintains muscle tone and decreases body fat. Produced in the ovaries and the adrenal glands in women and in the testes in men.	Low levels can cause decrease in libido, muscle mass and energy, increase in depression and the risk of osteoporosis.	Testosterone can increase within 20 minutes of intense exercise. Do lift heavy weights, exercise regularly, eat a diet rich in monounsaturated fats, get adequate sleep and limit alcohol. Try to control stress levels.

Hormone	Function	Imbalances	How to balance
Estrogen	Secreted by the ovaries, it is responsible for causing monthly ovulation. Can also increase fat breakdown from body stores. Elevates mood and libido.	Low levels can cause an increase in fat deposition in the abdominal region.	During menopause, the body reacts to the loss of estrogen from the ovaries by trying to produce more estrogen from fat cells. To make estrogen, the cells have to store more fat, which leads to weight gain. Regular exercise and a balanced diet can help.
Progesterone	Produced in the ovaries, it prepares the body for pregnancy. The precursor to many hormones, including estrogen and testosterone.	Low levels can cause water retention, bloating and an increase in weight.	For menopausal women, natural progesterone creams can be applied topically to help balance estrogen levels.
Leptin (the "fullness" hormone)	Secreted by fat cells, it tells the body when it is full (i.e., it's an appetite suppressant of sorts).	Low levels can cause an increase in food cravings and the desire to eat more.	Get adequate sleep and eat a diet rich in essential fats and proper proteins. Low leptin levels may also be linked to a zinc deficiency.

Hormone	Function	Imbalances	How to balance
Ghrelin	Secreted by the stomach, it increases hunger, slows metabolism and decreases the body's ability to burn fat. Levels increase during times of stress.	High levels can cause voracious hunger and trigger binge eating and weight gain.	Getting adequate sleep can help to reduce ghrelin levels and therefore reduce hunger.
Serotonin	A neurotransmitter found in the brain and responsible for mood.	Low levels can cause depression, fatigue, irritability and the desire for sweets and refined carbohydrates.	Increase protein, exercise and reduce stress—heightened cortisol can lower serotonin levels.
T4, the primary hormone converted to T3, the most active of the thyroid hormones	Produced by the thyroid gland, it raises metabolic rate.	Low levels can cause hypothyroidism. Symptoms include fatigue, a sluggish metabolism and weight gain.	Take synthetic or natural thyroid medications (prescribed by your doctor) and/or supplements (e.g., iodine; selenium; zinc; vitamins D, C and E; and essential fatty acids) as recommended by a natural practitioner.

Hormone	Function	Imbalances	How to balance
Growth hormone (GH)	Secreted by the pituitary gland, it decreases use of glucose and increases usage of fat. Primarily secreted during deepest phase of sleep.	Low levels can cause weight gain around the abdomen, depression, lack of energy and muscle wasting.	Release of growth hormone from the pituitary gland is greater with increasing aerobic exercise time, especially more intense exercise, such as interval training. Avoid sleep deprivation and interrupted sleep.
Endorphins	Secreted from the pituitary gland, they decrease appetite and reduce tension and anxiety.	Low levels can cause depression, fatigue and increase in pain levels.	Endorphins increase up to five times during longer aerobic exercise (30 minutes or longer). Listen to music, do something that thrills you, to increase endorphins.

For a detailed list of supplements that can help to balance hormones during menopause and supplements for adrenal health, see Appendix 5.

COMMON HORMONAL HEALTH ISSUES AND WEIGHT LOSS

In the same way that you can stimulate your hormones for weight loss, certain hormonal issues can sabotage your weight loss efforts. If you suspect you may be suffering from one of the health concerns outlined below, consult your doctor to discuss proper testing and diagnosis.

Type 2 diabetes

Type 2 diabetes (non-insulin-dependent diabetes) is a metabolic

> The glycated hemoglobin (HbA1c) test is commonly used as an indicator of how well a person has controlled their diabetes over the previous three months. Low-GI diets have been shown to lower HbA1c.

disorder and the most common form of diabetes. In short, type 2 diabetes affects how the body utilizes its glucose (sugar). People with type 2 diabetes tend to have high blood sugar because of insulin insensitivity. In other words, the cellular receptors begin to "ignore" their own insulin, becoming insulin insensitive. When this occurs, the pancreas is triggered to secrete more and more insulin to deal with the sugar from food. Excess insulin secretion leads to fat storage around the abdomen (resulting in an apple body shape). Eventually, the pancreas will conk out and stop producing insulin, and insulin drug therapy may be necessary. Approximately 90% of people with type 2 diabetes are overweight or obese. Type 2 diabetes is typically a reversible health condition with the proper dietary and lifestyle changes. The Metabolism Boosting Diet details specifics to lose weight, reduce insulin and maintain blood sugar control through food. Of course, it is advisable to talk to your doctor before beginning any new dietary plan.

Elevated cortisol and adrenal fatigue

In today's fast-paced, high-stress world, when we are faced with stressful situations, our body relies upon our adrenal glands (which sit atop the kidneys) to monitor our fight-or-flight response.

During times of stress, our adrenal glands respond by releasing two hormones: adrenaline, which makes us more alert, and cortisol, which converts protein to energy and releases our stored sugar, called glycogen. The glycogen becomes an instant source of fuel that we can utilize. When the stressful situation passes, the body quickly returns adrenaline levels to normal. Unfortunately, cortisol is not restored as quickly.

In prehistoric times, our stress response was based on short spurts of intense adrenaline release, as when we are chased by a bear. Luckily, in modern times, we do not normally have sudden bursts of such intense stress where we are running for our lives. Instead, the stress that most of us experience on a daily basis is in the form of mild to moderate swings throughout the day. This triggers cortisol secretion in the body. Surprisingly, short-term bouts of extreme high stress are actually healthier than long-term mild to moderate stress. The chronic nature of today's stress (running around with the kids, meeting deadlines, feeling rushed) creates the perfect environment for adrenal fatigue, which leads to weight gain.

Signs and symptoms of adrenal fatigue include weight gain, fatigue, insomnia, mental fogginess, depression, cravings and mood swings. It is important to keep in mind that the hormones insulin and cortisol are best friends, so to speak. In other words, when cortisol levels are up due to chronic stress, insulin levels will be driven up as well, making it harder to maintain blood sugar balance and support the body's fat-burning ability. This is why when my clients ask me, "What does stress have to do with weight gain?" my response is always, "Everything!"

If you suspect you may have elevated cortisol levels, which can lead to adrenal fatigue, talk to a natural health care practitioner or doctor about testing urine, blood or saliva levels of cortisol. Ideally, cortisol levels are high in the morning to give you energy and drop off near the evening so you can drift into a peaceful, restorative sleep. In the early stages of adrenal disruption, cortisol levels are too high during the day and continue rising into the evening. Eventually, just as the pancreas conks out and stops secreting normal amounts of insulin, the adrenal glands will become fatigued and will not produce enough of the necessary hormones for overall health and wellness. Keep in mind that shift work also can alter cortisol levels.

Hypothyroidism

Hypothyroidism is a condition characterized by abnormally low thyroid hormone production. The thyroid is one of the "master" glands that has an influence over metabolism and health. The two most important thyroid hormones are thyroxine (T4) and triiodothyronine (T3), which respectively account for 99% and 1% of thyroid hormones present in the blood. The production of these hormones is linked to a huge feedback loop and is stimulated by the pituitary gland, which in turn is regulated by the hypothalamus' thyrotropin-releasing hormone (TRH). In other words, the release of TRH from the hypothalamus tells the pituitary gland to release thyroid-stimulating hormones (TSHs). Any disruption in this feedback loop can create an insufficiency of thyroid hormones. The system works like this:

Hypothalamus (TRH) ⟶ Pituitary (TSH) ⟶ Thyroid (T4 and T3)

Hypothyroidism is a common condition. It is estimated that 3% to 5% of the population has some form of hypothyroidism. The most common type is an inherited condition called Hashimoto's thyroiditis, in which the thyroid gland is usually enlarged (i.e., a goitre) and has a decreased ability to make thyroid hormones. Hashimoto's is an autoimmune disease in which the body's immune system inappropriately attacks the thyroid tissue. The condition is more common in women than in men, and its incidence increases with age. Symptoms of hypothyroidism include modest weight gain, coarse hair, dry skin, constipation, excessive aches and pains, cold intolerance and extreme fatigue. Once tested and detected, hypothyroidism is typically treated with medication. Once treated, those diagnosed with hypothyroidism can lose weight just as well as any other healthy individual. It is important to note that no one single laboratory test diagnoses hypothyroidism 100%. It typically takes a combination of two or more tests to determine an abnormality.

Polycystic ovarian syndrome (PCOS)

Polycystic ovarian syndrome, or PCOS, is caused by an imbalance in the hormones (the chemical messengers) in a woman's brain and ovaries. Oftentimes, those with PCOS have heightened insulin levels, which result in excess testosterone production by the ovaries. Symptoms of PCOS can include weight gain, irregular periods, facial hair growth, difficulty losing weight, acne and infertility. According to an Australian study, even a modest amount of weight loss will help women with PCOS ovulate on a regular basis. In this study, 60 of 67 women with PCOS resumed ovulation after losing anywhere from 8 to 33 pounds (3.5 to 15 kg). In my clinical experience, women with PCOS have responded incredibly well to the dietary guidelines outlined in the Metabolism Boosting Diet.

Recently, two close friends, Janet and Ophelia, sought out my help for weight loss. Both women were in their mid-30s and had been diagnosed with PCOS, with a significant amount of weight to lose. When filling out their health history forms, they reported being frustrated with attempted weight loss plans in the past, which made them feel that, because of their PCOS, they were destined to be overweight for life. When reviewing their previous dietary approaches, it was clear to me that the women had been following a very strict "calories in, calories out" regimen that would never work long term thanks to their PCOS. Furthermore, their intake of monounsaturated fats and essential fatty acids (EFAs—fats that are critical to proper hormonal functioning) were critically low. Now, eager to finally gain control of their weight and feel their very best, they wanted to try again.

> Excess fat deposited in the abdominal region is often called "toxic fat," as it is strongly correlated to an increase in cardiovascular problems such as heart attacks and strokes.

From the get-go, it was obvious that both Janet and Ophelia required a plan that regulated blood sugars (and insulin) and provided them with sufficient caloric intake. In fact, with their previous dietary approaches, they were eating too little, which was causing feelings of hunger, cravings and deprivation. After putting them both on a hormonally balanced meal plan and suggesting certain supplements that would help boost their metabolism and balance their blood sugars, I am happy to report that Janet has lost over 71 pounds and Ophelia has lost more than 30 pounds!

THE BIG M—MENOPAUSE

I could not in good conscience put peri-menopause (the period before menopause where menstruation is irregular) or menopause in the category of health issues because they should *not* be categorized as a condition. Menopause is a natural time in a woman's life when the function of the ovaries ceases and menstruation stops. This transition can affect women in very different ways. Some sail through menopause with a minimum of the classic symptoms—hot flashes, disrupted sleep, change in mood and weight gain. Others struggle quite a bit when they're peri-menopausal and menopausal and report that they just don't feel like themselves anymore.

The big question I am constantly asked is "Can I lose weight and maintain my waist circumference in a healthy zone once I become menopausal?" The answer is a resounding yes! The Metabolism Boosting Diet takes your stage of life into account and makes the necessary adjustments to ensure your success. If you follow the dietary plan outlined in the following chapters and engage in regular physical activity, you will notice that the pounds start to melt away. Like anyone else on the program, you'll need to focus on hormonal balance and health, quality calories and optimal digestion. Of course, as we age, we have to take greater notice of our diet and activity level—and I will show you exactly how to do that. For the top supplement and dietary recommendation for peri-menopause and menopause, see Appendix 5.

Once you begin the first phase of the Metabolism Boosting Diet, your hormones (primarily insulin and glucagon) will balance and "flip the switch" on your metabolic engine. You'll experience weight loss, extra energy and a sense of balance within 3 to 7 days if you follow the initial phase strictly. My clients often ask me, "How do I know that I am in hormonal balance with food?" Trust me, you'll know. The difference in the way you feel is so dramatic—physically and emotionally—you'll wonder how you were ever functioning at full speed before. Other tangible markers include weight loss around the midsection (belly fat), a lack of cravings, the return of that "get up and go" energy that you perhaps thought was gone for good, and the return of an overall sense of daily well-being.

CORE ELEMENT #2: QUALITY CALORIES

Some people believe that weight loss is simply a function of mathematics. In other words, if you count calories in and calories out

SWITCH UP YOUR FAT

Studies have shown that simply switching types of fat can make a difference in weight loss. In one study, saturated fat was replaced with healthy monounsaturated fat (e.g., olive oil) for one group, while calories stayed the same in both groups. The participants who consumed the monounsaturated fat showed a significant improvement in insulin sensitivity, thereby promoting weight loss and disease prevention. Although calories stayed the same, simply switching the types of fat made a difference in blood sugar control and therefore weight loss.

and you are in a deficit, you will lose weight. But weight loss has to do with a lot more than just counting calories. The *quality* of the calories you are counting and consuming has a tremendous impact on your weight loss success. Take person A, for example, who is limiting her caloric intake to a modest 1,200 calories per day but is consuming a white bagel for breakfast, sugary coffees throughout the day and grabbing cookies for energy when experiencing the 3 p.m. slump. Will this individual lose weight as effectively as person B, who is eating 1,200 calories of healthy fats, lean proteins and low-GI carbohydrates? Of course not! In addition, person A will experience a far greater degree of lethargy, will clog her digestive pipes from her faulty nutrition and will run the risk of developing poor blood sugar control, high cholesterol and type 2 diabetes.

Of course, when we are discussing calories, we must keep the *quantity* of calories we are consuming in mind also. There is a balance between eating too many calories and eating too few. There is a very popular weight loss program on the market that promotes extreme caloric restriction (a mere 600 calories per day). Of course, initial weight loss will occur (and a lot of water loss as well), but when you pose the question raised at the beginning of the book—"Can I see myself following a version of this program in 5 years' time?"—the answer is an absolute no. Although people following extreme caloric restriction lose an abundant amount of weight, this weight loss is temporary and unsustainable. Usually, one of two common scenarios plays out:

1. A person on a severe calorie-restricted diet goes to a special event or party, or simply becomes fed up with the diet, and starts food binging. Within a very short time, he quickly packs on 5, 10 or 15 pounds, which begins the vicious unhealthy weight loss cycle: feeling beat up and distraught, he throws all his attempts to lose weight out the window and gives in to his cravings, which quickly come rushing back. The lure of rapid weight loss seemed appealing at the time; now it is creating feelings of defeat and frustration. I have seen clients binge eat and gain back 6 to 8 pounds within a week following extreme caloric restriction.

2. An individual who is consuming too few calories enters a physical state known as "starvation adaptation mode," where the body becomes extremely efficient at storing calories as fat. Behaving as though it is in a time of starvation, the body stores every precious calorie as fat for future fuel in a mistaken effort to protect the brain and the internal organs. This is why people who come off extreme calorie-restricted diets tend at first to experience a sluggishness in their metabolic capacity. (Fear not, this can be turned around by including the proper fats, proteins and carbohydrates into the mix to fuel the metabolic engine once again.)

Eventually, for those on an calorie-restricted diet, the body rebels because of low energy, fatigue, constipation or other complications, and its need for a more balanced approach takes over.

On the flip side, the other issue we have in North America is eating too many calories. The two-for-one, bigger-is-better, supersize-me attitude has created a population where over two-thirds are overweight or obese. Typical dinner plate sizes have actually increased in restaurants from 10 to 12 inches, sugar consumption is at an all-time high and food additives such as MSG (monosodium glutamate) trick the brain into consuming more and more. The key is to find the balance between not eating too many calories and not eating too few.

In all the areas of research in the nutritional world, the most promising results in human and animal studies involve mild caloric restriction, which has been shown to increase life span significantly and decrease age-related disease processes. Before you panic, I must stress the word *mild.* Unlike the extreme caloric restriction diets of 600 calories per day, mild caloric restriction means a 15% to 20% reduction in calories per day. The average North American consumes 2,100 to 2,500 calories each day. If this is lowered by 15%, that is a reduction of approximately 315 to 375 calories per day. In the initial stages of the Metabolism Boosting Diet, the caloric restriction will be slightly more, but you will not feel hungry, nor will you ever drop below 1,000 calories a day. When following the Metabolism Boosting Diet plan, the *quality* of the calories you are eating (from fibre, fat, protein and slow-burning carbohydrates) will fill you up and expand in your stomach; thus, you will quickly notice that you eat less but are completely free of cravings and hunger. Once you hit the MAINTENANCE stage, your caloric intake will rise without altering your weight. Your set point will have changed, and you will easily be able to enjoy a variety of foods and beverages without unwanted weight gain. If you are highly active, that too will be taken into account and your caloric intake will be increased.

CORE ELEMENT #3: DIGESTIVE CAPACITY

As I mentioned earlier, "You are only as healthy as your pipes" is one of my key statements. In other words, you are only as healthy as you are efficient at digesting, absorbing and excreting. If your "pipes" do not function adequately and eliminate on a daily basis, weight loss can be sluggish and frustrating. Along with that, uncomfortable symptoms can develop, from constipation and malabsorption of nutrients to fatigue, headaches, bloating, water retention, acid reflux, joint and muscle pain, sugar cravings and skin breakouts.

HOW WELL ARE YOU DIGESTING?

Take the tape measure test to see how well you are digesting. Measure your waist circumference in your belly button region first thing in the morning, before eating your first meal. Then take your measurement in the evening before going to bed. If your waist circumference has increased more than 1 to 2 inches from morning to evening, it may be a sign that you are not properly digesting or eliminating your food.

Another important element associated with optimal digestion is the digestive-food-mood link. Most people are by now familiar with the neurotransmitter (brain chemical) called serotonin. If serotonin is deficient in the body, mild to severe symptoms of depression can develop. This is why so many people opt to take an SSRI (selective serotonin re-uptake inhibitor—Prozac is one such medication). SSRIs ensure more serotonin is circulating in your brain to help alleviate feelings of depression.

So you may ask, what does this have to do with digestion? Well, what most people are not aware of is that 95% of our serotonin is produced in the gut. In fact, the gut has often been referred to as our "second brain." I am confident that research, when it catches up, will show that a healthy gut lining and supplementation with probiotics ("good" bacteria) will offer substantial promise for mood disorders, depression and weight loss. I can tell you, based on my clinical experience, that the healthier one's digestive functioning, the better one feels both mentally and physically and the more weight one tends to lose overall. Or, as the writer Sydney Smith once remarked, "I am convinced digestion is the great secret to life."

THE BODY'S ORCHESTRA

The body comprises several systems, including the cardiovascular, lymphatic, respiratory and endocrine. The totality of the systems can be likened to that of an orchestra. When all instruments are in tune and at their best, the piece of music flows beautifully without a note ever being off-key. But if one of the instruments is off—say it has not been taken care of properly and needs tuning or cleaning—it will affect the entire song.

Similarly, when the digestive system is off for whatever reason—maybe from consuming too many processed foods, eating too much, a lack of fibre, dehydration or stress—many other bodily systems may be affected. Some people may not make the link, but faulty digestion and absorption can indeed create myriad health complaints and, if not taken care of, can lead to serious diseases. Although there is no one master system that runs the body—all are equally important—the digestive system has an enormous impact on how you feel, look and function on a daily basis.

THE FUNDAMENTALS OF DIGESTION

The digestive system is made up of the mouth, pharynx, esophagus, stomach, small intestine, large intestine (also called the colon) rectum and anus. To help us understand the basics of digestion and how other bodily systems are involved, let's consider a sample scenario. Suppose you eat a chicken wrap for lunch. Digestion really begins when you simply smell the sandwich, which triggers nerves in the brain to respond by salivating (thus the term *mouth-watering*). Following that, the process works in this way:

1. You take the first bite of the sandwich, which causes even more saliva to be secreted, aiding in the breakdown of the food. When the food is in your mouth, an enzyme called amylase is secreted to begin carbohydrate digestion.

2. Once chewed, the food slides down your pharynx to the esophagus, which leads directly into the stomach. Once the food is in the stomach, an involuntary muscle contraction known as peristalsis begins to churn the food.

HEARTBURN

Have you ever experienced heartburn? At the end of the esophagus, the lower esophageal sphincter lets the food into the stomach. It opens and then quickly closes to keep the food from escaping back into the esophagus. Heartburn occurs when this sphincter isn't working properly and stomach acid manages to splash into the esophagus. If this happens chronically, you might have gastroesophageal reflux disease. Eating a low-acid diet (free of white sugar, pop, deep-fried foods and coffee), drinking plenty of water, chewing your food well and supplementing with ginger, aloe vera and digestive enzymes can help tremendously.

3. Glands in the stomach secrete an acid, while enzymes and a mucosal layer protect the stomach from its own acidic secretion. The acid secretion in the stomach is necessary to break down the food in preparation for its next stop, the small intestine. By the time your bite of sandwich leaves your stomach, it is in a liquid form known as chyme.
4. Once the chyme is in the small intestine, absorption begins. The small intestine is made up of three parts: the duodenum, jejunum and ileum. The small intestine is covered by millions of projections called villi, which are integral for absorption. The villi "grab" nutrients from the chyme that was once your sandwich and move it through the wall of the intestinal tract into the blood vessels, to be transported throughout the body. Once all the "good stuff" has been taken from the food, the indigestible parts are transported to the large intestine for excretion.
5. The large intestine is the last stop of the digestive process. The large intestine absorbs extra fluid to produce the solid waste called feces.

The digestive tract has other "helpers" that assist with digestion, including glands, hormones, nerves and organs. The *glands* that help out are:

- ***the liver***—helps in digesting and absorbing fats by secreting bile. The bile is made in the liver and secreted through bile ducts into the small intestine.
- ***the gall bladder***—acts as a "warehouse" for extra bile.
- ***the pancreas***—secretes pancreatic juices filled with enzymes that are necessary for optimal digestion.

The main *hormones* involved in the digestive process are:

- ***gastrin***—signals the stomach to produce acid to aid in food absorption.

- ***secretin***—triggers the pancreas to send out a digestive juice that is rich in bicarbonate, which helps to neutralize stomach acids as they enter the small intestine. Secretin also stimulates the stomach to secrete pepsin, which is responsible for protein digestion and stimulates the liver to secrete bile.
- ***CCK***—stimulates the pancreas to secrete pancreatic juices and stimulates the gall bladder to empty.
- ***ghrelin***—produced in the stomach and upper intestinal tract and stimulates appetite.
- ***peptide YY***—produced in the stomach and upper intestinal tract and has been shown to inhibit appetite.
- ***leptin***—a fat-derived hormone that has also been shown to inhibit appetite. Some research indicates that obese individuals can develop a resistance to leptin.

The main *nerves* that assist with digestion are:

- ***extrinsic nerves***—found in the unconscious part of the brain and spinal cord, they work by stimulating the release of the chemicals acetylcholine and adrenaline. Acetylcholine stimulates hormones to make digestive juices in the stomach and pancreas. The other critical role of acetylcholine is to cause the muscles of the digestive tract to contract and move food along. Adrenaline has an opposing role, relaxing muscles of the digestive system when there is no food.
- ***intrinsic nerves***—found within the digestive system, from the esophagus to the colon. These nerves are not signalled by the brain but are triggered when food stretches out the walls of the digestive system. Depending on the amount of food consumed, these nerves either speed up or slow down digestion.

As you can see, the process of digestion is extremely sophisticated, involving glands, hormones, nerves and more. Thus, when your digestive capacity is compromised due to faulty food choices, mineral deficiencies, stress or dehydration, your health can suffer. This is also why you are truly only as healthy as your pipes and why the integrity of your digestive capacity is a fundamental part of your weight loss journey.

"I FEEL BLOATED"

Of all the complaints about digestion I encounter daily, one of the most common is the feeling of being bloated. There are numerous factors that may contribute to bloating, making you feel uncomfortable throughout the day. The most common causes of bloating include the following:

- water retention
- stress
- food intolerances (food sensitivities or allergies)
- overconsumption of foods (i.e., portion distortion—eating too much at one time)

HOW IS YOUR DIGESTIVE HEALTH?

- Do you have fewer than one bowel movement per day?
- Is your bowel movement strained?
- Does your waist circumference increase more than 1 to 2 inches from morning to evening?
- Do you constantly feel bloated or full?
- Do you rely on laxatives to go to the bathroom?
- Do you continually have acid reflux, belching or bad gas?
- Is your bowel movement formed (tip: bowel movements should float in the toilet bowl and be S- or C-shaped)
- Do you have bloating, distension or pain after eating a meal?
- Do you suffer from chronic yeast infections or have you been diagnosed with candida (yeast) in the past?

- deficiency in enzyme secretions
- irritable bowel syndrome

From a hormonal perspective, it is quite common for women to experience bloating the week before their menstruation. When this occurs, an excess amount of fluid builds up in the spaces between the cells. Associated symptoms may be swollen and puffy eyes, fingers or ankles.

If you feel you are experiencing water retention, a quick way to check is to press your thumb onto your calf for 5 to 10 seconds and then release the pressure. Does the skin spring back or is an indentation left? An indentation is often a sign of fluid retention, which may be affecting the number on your scale. If you are chronically experiencing symptoms of fluid retention, talk to your doctor.

DIGESTIVE TIPS TO HELP YOU ON YOUR WEIGHT LOSS JOURNEY

Along with the foods that are recommended as part of the Metabolism Boosting Diet, there are certain digestive behaviours that can help you lose weight more quickly and ensure that your "pipes" are in tiptop shape:

- Eat until you are sufficiently full, not stuffed. Your stomach needs room to properly digest the food you are eating. If you overconsume, you will tax your digestive system, which can result in bloating, undigested food particles and poor digestion.
- Chew your food very well to ensure optimal digestion. You want your food to be in a paste form before swallowing to aid the digestive process. In addition, try to make your meals last as long as possible—20 minutes or longer is ideal.
- Drink water between and with meals to aid digestion.
- Start and finish your day with hot water and lemon juice.

Lemon is a natural astringent but is also helpful in breaking down food.

- If you think you may be sensitive to certain foods (dairy, gluten and wheat being the most common culprits), eliminate the suspected offending foods for a minimum of 2 weeks and watch for an improvement.
- Top-load your day with food. In other words, make dinner your smallest meal of the day. As you will see in the following chapter, supper is supplementary.
- Consider supplementing your meals with digestive enzymes (in capsule, chewable pill or liquid form).

You will find that once you start on the Metabolism Boosting Diet, your digestive capacity will increase and improve dramatically. The foods and meal plans outlined in the following chapters are rich in must-have foods that promote healthy elimination, detoxification and nourishment.

PART II
THE PLAN

CHAPTER 6

DETERMINE YOUR METABOLIC ID

We are indeed much more than what we eat, but what we eat can help us to become much more than whom we are.

—Adele Davis, nutrition pioneer

In the text that follows, you will find the Metabolic ID Questionnaire (there is one for women, another for men). Take the time to answer the questions as carefully as you can, choosing the answers that best fit your current situation and lifestyle. Your results will determine the length of time you will remain in the first phase of the program, the BALANCE phase. The Metabolic ID questionnaire is designed to take into account all about you—your age, eating habits, hormonal health, activity level, sleep patterns and emotional relationship with food. Once you have completed the questionnaire, tally up your score, refer to the legend at the end of this chapter and you are ready to begin!

METABOLIC ID QUESTIONNAIRE FOR WOMEN

ABOUT YOU

1. How much weight would you like to lose?

5 to 15 pounds (2.2 to 6.75 kg) = 1 point

16 to 30 pounds (7.25 to 13.5 kg) = 2 points

31 to 50 pounds (14 to 22.75 kg) = 3 points

> 50 pounds (> 22.75 kg) = 4 points

2. Measure your waist circumference (see page 43 for instructions). Is it greater than 35 inches (88 cm)?

Yes = 1 point

No = 0 points

3. How long have you struggled with your weight?

< 1 year = 0 points

1 year = 1 point

2 to 5 years = 2 points

> 5 years = 3 points

All my life = 4 points

4. Were you overweight as a child?

Yes = 1 point

No = 0 points

5. Are either of your parents or any of your siblings overweight?

Yes = 1 point

No = 0 points

6. What is your current level of stress on a daily basis?

I do not feel stressed = 0 points

Low = 1 point

Medium = 2 points

High = 3 points

Extremely high = 4 points

7. Do you often feel you have too many responsibilities and not enough time?

Yes = 1 point

No = 0 points

8. How often do you work out?

I do not work out = 3 points

1 time per week = 2 points

2 times per week = 1 point

3 to 5 times per week = 0 points

9. How long do you sit in front of a computer screen daily?

I do not sit in front of a computer screen = 0 points

1 to 2 hours per day = 1 point

2 to 4 hours per day = 2 points

4 to 6 hours per day = 3 points

6 to 8 hours per day = 4 points

10. Do you work a night shift position?

Yes = 4 points

No = 0 points

11. How long is your commute to work?

I don't commute to work = 0 points

Up to 1 hour each way = 1 point

> 1 hour each way = 2 points

12. Have you quit smoking within the last 6 months?

Yes = 2 points

No = 0 points

13. How frequent are your bowel movements?

Daily = 0 points

Every other day = 1 point

Every 2 to 3 days = 2 points

Every 4 to 5 days = 3 points

14. Do you feel bloated on a daily basis?

Yes = 2 points

No = 0 points

15. Do you often have trouble falling asleep?

Yes = 1 point

No = 0 points

16. Do you often wake up more than once at night?

Yes = 2 points

No = 0 points

17. Do you typically wake in the morning feeling rested?

Yes = 0 points

No = 1 point

18. Do you take a sleeping pill to help you fall asleep?

Yes = 1 point

No = 0 points

19. Are you on antidepressant medication?

Yes = 1 point

No = 0 points

20. What is your energy level like on a daily basis?

I have great energy = 0 points

My energy fluctuates throughout the day = 1 point

I have very low energy = 2 points

Total "About You" score = _____

YOUR EATING HABITS

21. Do you eat after dinner?

Yes = 3 points

No = 0 points

22. On a busy day, do you tend to skip meals?

Yes = 1 point

No = 0 points

23. When at social events, do you find it hard not to overindulge?

Yes = 1 point

No = 0 points

24. Do you often give in to sweets cravings?

Yes = 1 point

No = 0 points

25. Do you crave salt?

Yes = 1 point

No = 0 points

26. How many alcoholic drinks do you consume per week?

I do not drink alcohol = 0 points

2 drinks = 1 point

4 drinks = 2 points

6 drinks = 3 points

8 drinks = 4 points

10 drinks = 5 points

> 10 drinks = 6 points

27. How many cups of coffee do you drink per day?

0 to 1 cup = 0 points

2 cups = 1 point

2 to 4 cups = 2 points

> 4 cups = 3 points

28. How many 8-ounce (250 mL) glasses of water do you drink per day?

I do not drink water on a daily basis = 4 points

Up to 2 glasses = 3 points

2 to 4 glasses = 2 points

4 to 6 glasses = 1 point

6 to 8 glasses = 0 points

29. Have you been on a high-protein diet in the past 6 months?

Yes = 1 point

No = 0 points

30. Have you been on a calorie-restricted diet (fewer than 1,000 calories per day) in the past 6 months?

Yes = 1 point

No = 0 points

31. How often do you eat out?

Maximum once per week = 0 points

1 to 3 times per week = 1 point

3 to 5 times per week = 2 points

5 to 7 times per week = 3 points

32. How often do you eat fast food?

Rarely = 0 points

1 to 2 times per week = 1 point

2 to 4 times per week = 2 points

4 to 6 times per week = 3 points

Total "Your Eating Habits" Score: _____

YOUR HORMONAL HEALTH

33. Do you have irregular periods?

Yes = 1 point

No = 0 points

34. Are you peri- or post-menopausal?

Yes = 2 points

No = 0 points

35. Have you had a partial or full hysterectomy?

Yes = 2 points

No = 0 points

36. Have you been diagnosed with polycystic ovarian syndrome (PCOS)?

Yes = 2 points

No = 0 points

37. Have you been diagnosed with a thyroid condition?

Yes = 2 points

No = 0 points

38. Do you have hypoglycemia (low blood sugar)—do you feel shaky, irritable or moody if you skip a meal or snack?

Yes = 1 point

No = 0 points

39. Have you been diagnosed with type 2 diabetes?

Yes = 2 points

No = 0 points

40. Do you experience the 3 p.m. slump (i.e., tiredness mid-afternoon)?

Yes = 1 point

No = 0 points

41. Do you often feel tired after eating a meal?

Yes = 1 point

No = 0 points

Total "Your Hormonal Health" Score: ______

YOUR EMOTIONAL RELATIONSHIP WITH FOOD

42. Do you classify yourself as an emotional eater (you eat if you're happy, bored, sad, lonely)?

Yes = 1 point

No = 0 points

43. Do you find you usually start your day off eating healthy, only to end it in an unhealthy way?

Yes = 1 point

No = 0 points

44. Do you feel you have a healthy relationship with food?

Yes = 0 points

Sometimes = 1 point

No = 2 points

45. Do you think about your weight more than once per day?

Yes = 1 point

No = 0 points

46. When you "cheat" on a diet, do you feel as if you have blown the entire thing and end up doing more cheating or binging?

Yes = 1 point

No = 0 points

47. Do you feel guilty after you eat?

Yes = 2 points

Sometimes = 1 point

No = 0 points

48. Do you often eat alone?

Yes = 1 point

No = 0 points

49. When trying to lose weight in the past, did you find you were an "all or nothing" person—either following the diet 100% or falling off it completely?

Yes = 1 point

No = 0 points

50. Does your weight influence your overall mood on a daily basis?

No = 0 points

Occasionally = 1 point

Yes = 2 points

51. How much is your weight bothering you?

It does not bother me = 0 points

It bothers me moderately = 1 point

It bothers me significantly = 2 points

Total "Your Emotional Relationship with Food" Score: _____

TOTAL SCORES:

About You: _____

Your Eating Habits: _____

Your Hormonal Health: _____

Your Emotional Relationship with Food: _____

GRAND TOTAL:_____

SCORING ANALYSIS FOR WOMEN

0 TO 30 POINTS—5 DAYS IN THE BALANCE PHASE

If you scored 30 or below, enter Phase 1—BALANCE—for 5 days. Your score indicates that you likely have a relatively small amount of weight to lose and possess a fairly good metabolic capacity. You likely have not struggled with your weight for a long period and were not overweight as a child. While you may experience a degree of cravings or faulty eating patterns, your score indicates that these patterns are relatively minor and that you require only some metabolic fine tuning to get you to your goal weight. Your time in the BALANCE phase will help you to obtain proper blood sugar control to ensure you quickly enter a fat-burning mode. You will find that your cravings for sweets, alcohol and/or salt will be completely eliminated by the time you have completed the BALANCE phase, and you will notice a surge in energy and vitality. Since you do not have that much weight to lose, you will quickly notice a flattening and strengthening in the abdominal region, and any degree of bloating should also disappear upon completion of the BALANCE phase.

31 TO 60 POINTS—10 DAYS IN THE BALANCE PHASE

If you scored between 31 and 60, enter Phase 1—BALANCE—for 10 days. Your score indicates that you likely have 15 to 40 pounds (6.75 to 18 kg) to lose and that in the past you have struggled with your weight to a certain degree. You may be an emotional eater who tends to crave sweet food and indulges at night. Like so many others, chances are you start your day in a very healthy fashion, only to complete it in an unhealthy manner (e.g., nighttime eating, dining out, too much alcohol). You may also have a hormonal underlay (menopause or a thyroid issue, say) or a current stressful event that is elevating your cortisol levels and causing you to store fat in your abdominal region. It is also likely that you have more of an apple body shape than a pear body shape, with a waist circumference of more than 35 inches (88 cm). The BALANCE phase is designed to jumpstart your metabolic set point and to maximize fat and inch loss. After 10 days in this phase, you will quickly notice flattening around your midsection and will feel far less bloated and more energetic. While your cravings may heighten in the first 1 to 3 days of the BALANCE phase, they will quickly subside and become a thing of the past. Improvement in sleep and a decrease in nighttime sweating are also frequently noticed when in the BALANCE phase for this length of time. Use the Metabolism Boosting Tracking Chart, found on page 272, to monitor your progress.

61 TO 100 POINTS—15 DAYS IN THE BALANCE PHASE

If you scored between 61 and 100, enter Phase 1—BALANCE—for 15 days. Your score indicates that you have a significant amount of weight to lose (likely more than 50 lbs/22.75 kgs), have struggled with your weight for several years and likely have emotional eating patterns (e.g., using food to soothe or binge eating at night). You may have also been overweight as a child or have had a sibling or a parent who is also overweight. Your weight loss journey will begin with the BALANCE phase for 15 days. You have likely tried several diets in the past, so it is critical to ensure your blood sugars are normalized to maximize the fat-burning effect and rev your metabolism. You will know that you are implementing the BALANCE phase properly when you no longer feel hungry, are crave-free and are feeling a significant increase in energy and mood. You should also feel far more control over your food choices and not feel the need to binge eat or "cheat." For maximum effectiveness and to put an end to emotional eating patterns, it is strongly recommended that you utilize the Metabolism Boosting Food Journal, a sample of which is found on page 271, to record your food intake and your moods on a daily basis. Do not focus on the total amount of weight you have to lose—you will get there! Focus instead on 10 pounds

(4.5 kg) at a time, and before you know it, you will be at your goal weight and feel fitter, healthier, leaner and stronger.

METABOLIC ID QUESTIONNAIRE FOR MEN

ABOUT YOU

1. How much weight would you like to lose?

5 to 15 pounds (2.2 to 6.75 kg) = 1 point

16 to 30 pounds (7.25 to 13.5 kg) = 2 points

31 to 50 pounds (14 to 22.75 kg) = 3 points

> 50 pounds (22.75 kg) = 4 points

2. Measure your waist circumference (see page 43 for instructions). Is it greater than 40 inches (102 cm)?

Yes = 1 point

No = 0 points

3. How long have you struggled with your weight?

> 1 year = 0 points

1 year = 1 point

2 to 5 years = 2 points

> 5 years = 3 points

All my life = 4 points

4. Were you overweight as a child?

Yes = 1 point

No = 0 points

5. Are either of your parents or any of your siblings overweight?

Yes = 1 point

No = 0 points

6. What is your current level of stress on a daily basis?

I do not feel stressed = 0 points

Low = 1 point

Medium = 2 points

High = 3 points

Extremely high = 4 points

7. Do you often feel you have too many responsibilities and not enough time?

Yes = 1 point

No = 0 points

8. How often do you work out?

I do not work out = 3 points

1 time per week = 2 points

2 times per week = 1 point

3 to 5 times per week = 0 points

9. How long do you sit in front of a computer screen daily?

I do not sit in front of a computer screen = 0 points

1 to 2 hours per day = 1 point

2 to 4 hours per day = 2 points

4 to 6 hours per day = 3 points

6 to 8 hours per day = 4 points

10. Do you work a night shift position?

Yes = 4 points

No = 0 points

11. How long is your commute to work?

I don't commute to work = 0 points

Up to 1 hour each way = 1 point

> 1 hour each way = 2 points

12. Have you quit smoking within the past 6 months?

Yes = 2 points

No = 0 points

13. How frequent are your bowel movements?

Daily = 0 points

Every other day = 1 point

Every 2 to 3 days = 2 points

Every 4 to 5 days = 3 points

14. Do you feel bloated on a daily basis?

Yes = 2 points

No = 0 points

15. Do you often have trouble falling asleep?

Yes = 1 point

No = 0 points

16. Do you often wake up more than once at night?

Yes = 2 points

No = 0 points

17. Do you typically wake up in the morning feeling rested?

Yes = 0 points

No = 1 point

18. Do you take a sleeping pill to help you fall asleep?

Yes = 1 point

No = 0 points

19. Are you on antidepressant medication?

Yes = 1 point

No = 0 points

20. What is your energy level like on a daily basis?

I have great energy = 0 points

My energy fluctuates throughout the day = 1 point

I have very low energy = 2 points

Total "About You" Score = ______

YOUR EATING HABITS

21. Do you eat after dinner?

Yes = 3 points

No = 0 points

22. On a busy day, do you tend to skip meals?

Yes = 1 point

No = 0 points

23. When at social events, do you find it hard not to overindulge?

Yes = 1 point

No = 0 points

24. Do you often give in to sweets cravings?

Yes = 1 point

No = 0 points

25. Do you crave salt?

Yes = 1 point

No = 0 points

26. How many alcoholic drinks do you consume per week?

I do not drink alcohol = 0 points

2 drinks = 1 point

4 drinks = 2 points

6 drinks = 3 points

8 drinks = 4 points

10 drinks = 5 points

> 10 drinks = 6 points

27. How many cups of coffee do you drink per day?

0 to 1 cup = 0 points

2 cups = 1 point

2 to 4 cups = 2 points

> 4 cups = 3 points

28. How many 8 ounce (250 mL) glasses of water do you drink per day?

I do not drink water on a daily basis = 4 points

Up to 2 glasses = 3 points

2 to 4 glasses = 2 points

4 to 6 glasses = 1 point

6 to 8 glasses = 0 points

29. Have you been on a high-protein diet in the past 6 months?

Yes = 1 point

No = 0 points

30. Have you been on a calorie-restricted diet (fewer than 1,000 calories per day) in the past 6 months?

Yes = 1 point

No = 0 points

31. How often do you dine out?

Maximum once per week = 0 points

1 to 3 times per week = 1 point

3 to 5 times per week = 2 points

5 to 7 times per week = 3 points

32. How often do you eat fast food?

Rarely = 0 points

1 to 2 times per week = 1 point

2 to 4 times per week = 2 points

4 to 6 times per week = 3 points

Total "Your Eating Habits" Score: _____

YOUR HORMONAL HEALTH

33. Do you experience any symptoms of andropause (defined as the lowering of testosterone with aging; symptoms include irritability, low sex drive and fatigue)?

Yes = 3 points

No = 0 points

34. Are you over 55?

Yes = 2 points

No = 0 points

35. Have you noticed a significant loss of muscle strength in the last 6 months?

Yes = 2 points

No = 0 points

36. Have you been diagnosed with a thyroid condition?

Yes = 2 points

No = 0 points

37. Do you have hypoglycemia (low blood sugar)—do you feel shaky, irritable or moody if you skip a meal or snack?

Yes = 1 point

No = 0 points

38. Have you been diagnosed with type 2 diabetes?

Yes = 2 points

No = 0 points

39. Do you experience the 3 p.m. slump (i.e., tiredness mid-afternoon)?

Yes = 1 point

No = 0 points

40. Do you often feel tired after eating a meal?

Yes = 1 point

No = 0 points

Total "Your Hormonal Health" Score: _____

YOUR EMOTIONAL RELATIONSHIP WITH FOOD

41. Do you classify yourself as an emotional eater (you eat if you're happy, bored, sad, lonely)?

Yes = 1 point

No = 0 points

42. Do you find you usually start your day off eating healthy, only to end it in an unhealthy way?

Yes = 1 point

No = 0 points

43. Do you feel you have a healthy relationship with food?

Yes = 0 points

Sometimes = 1 point

No = 2 points

44. Do you think about your weight more than once per day?

Yes = 1 point

No = 0 points

45. When you "cheat" on a diet, do you feel as if you have blown the entire thing and end up doing more cheating or binging?

Yes = 1 point

No = 0 points

46. Do you feel guilty after you eat?

Yes = 2 points

Sometimes = 1 point

No = 0 points

47. Do you often eat alone?

Yes = 1 point

No = 0 points

48. When trying to lose weight in the past, did you find you were an "all or nothing" person—either following the diet 100% or falling off it completely?

Yes = 1 point

No = 0 points

49. Does your weight influence your overall mood on a daily basis?

No = 0 points

Occasionally = 1 point

Yes = 2 points

50. How much is your weight bothering you?

It does not bother me = 0 points

It bothers me moderately = 1 point

It bothers me significantly = 2 points

Total "Your Emotional Relationship with Food" Score: _____

TOTAL SCORES

About You: _____

Your Eating Habits: _____

Your Hormonal Health: _____

Your Emotional Relationship with Food: _____

GRAND TOTAL: _____

SCORING ANALYSIS FOR MEN

0 TO 30 POINTS—5 DAYS IN THE BALANCE PHASE

If you scored 30 or below, enter Phase 1—BALANCE—for 5 days. Your score indicates that you likely have a relatively small amount of weight to lose and possess a fairly good metabolic capacity. Between life, work and stress, a small amount of weight has likely crept up on you, and it is time to take care of it. You likely have not struggled with your weight for a long period and were not overweight as a child. While you may experience a degree of cravings or faulty eating patterns, your score indicates that these are minor and that you require some metabolic fine tuning to reach your goal weight. Your time in the BALANCE phase will help you to obtain proper blood sugar control to ensure you quickly enter a fat-burning mode. Men have a stronger metabolic and fat-burning capacity overall than women, so your time in the BALANCE phase to obtain maximum results will be short and sweet. You will find that your cravings for sugar, alcohol and/or salt will be completely eliminated by the time you have completed the BALANCE phase, and you will notice a surge in energy and vitality. Since you do not have that much weight to lose, you will quickly notice a flattening and strengthening in the abdominal region, and any degree of bloating should also disappear upon completion of the BALANCE phase.

31 TO 60 POINTS—10 DAYS IN BALANCE PHASE

If you scored between 31 and 60, enter Phase 1—BALANCE—for 10 days. Your score indicates that you likely have 15 to 40 pounds (6.75 to 18 kg) to lose and that in the past you have struggled with your weight to a certain degree. Your weight gain is likely due to a mix of lack of activity, eating too late, a high-stress job, too many sweets or alcohol and faulty food choices. Like so many other men, you are likely storing your weight in your abdominal region (i.e., you have an apple body shape), which increases your risk for cardiovascular disease, the development of high cholesterol and stroke. The good news is, for every 5 pounds (2.2 kg) you lose, you will lose 1 inch (2.5 cm) or more from your waistline. The BALANCE phase is designed to jumpstart your metabolic set point and maximize fat and inch loss. After 10 days in this phase, you will quickly notice flattening around your midsection and will feel far less bloated and more energetic. While your cravings may heighten in the first 1 to 3 days of the BALANCE phase, they will quickly subside and become a thing of the past. Improvement in sleep and a decrease in snoring and nighttime sweating is also frequently noticed when in the BALANCE phase for this length of time. Use the Metabolism Boosting Tracking Chart, found on page 272, to monitor your progress.

61 TO 100 POINTS—15 DAYS IN BALANCE PHASE

If you scored between 61 and 100, enter Phase 1—BALANCE—for 15 days. Your score indicates that you have a significant amount of weight to lose (likely more than 50 lb/22.75 kg). You may have gained your weight due to fast food, excessive alcohol, stress, travel or nighttime eating. The weight is likely impacting your activity level, mood and overall health. Your weight loss journey will begin with the BALANCE phase for 15 days. The length of time you will spend in the BALANCE phase is designed to balance your blood sugars and boost your metabolic potential. You have likely tried several diets in the past, so it is critical to ensure your blood sugars are normalized to maximize the fat-burning effect and rev your metabolism. You will know that you are implementing the BALANCE phase properly when you no longer feel hungry, are crave-free and are feeling a significant increase in energy and mood. You should also feel far more control over your food choices and not feel the need to binge eat or "cheat." Best of all, in this phase weight loss will be fast and noticeable. For maximum effectiveness and to put an end to emotional eating patterns, it is strongly recommended that you utilize the Metabolism Boosting Food Journal, a sample of which is found on page 271, to record your food intake and your mood on a daily basis. Do not focus on the total amount of weight you have to lose—you will get there! Focus on 10 pounds (4.5 kg) at a time and before you know it, you will be at your goal weight and feel fitter, healthier, leaner and stronger.

CHAPTER 7

PHASE 1: BALANCE

There is no try, only do.
—Yoda, from *Star Wars*

The purpose of the BALANCE phase is to stabilize blood sugar and hormone levels, which initiates the process of fat-burning, especially in the abdominal region. This will also be the part of the program that puts an end to your intense sweet cravings, which ultimately lead to poor food choices and food binging patterns. I strongly believe that in order to effectively address faulty eating patterns (e.g., emotional eating, food binging, nighttime eating), it is critical to, first and foremost, follow the dietary plan outlined below. Once you are in control of your blood sugars and obtain hormonal balance, you can better deal with your emotional eating patterns. In short, balance first, shift and change emotional eating patterns second—you can't win if you are craving sugar!

BENEFITS OF THE BALANCE PHASE

The benefits of this phase include balanced blood sugars, reduced insulin levels, fat-burning effects in the abdominal region initiated and cravings eliminated. This phase also promotes cleansing and digestive health.

LENGTH OF THE BALANCE PHASE

Depending on your score on the Metabolic ID Questionnaire, this phase will last 5, 10 or 15 days. Because you are in the BALANCE phase for only a short period, it is important to stick to the dietary plan as strictly as you possibly can. Once you have completed the determined length of time in this phase, you will have more leeway and variety as far as food choices go. More grains, treats and alcohol options will come, in moderation—just be patient and get balanced first.

Along with an outline of the structure of your daily meals and snacks, in this chapter you will find a list of:

- "free" foods—those you can eat as much of as you like
- limited foods
- foods that will cut cravings
- no-no foods—foods not permitted at this stage

You'll also find a 7-Day BALANCE Meal Plan and easy-to-make recipes that will make life a little easier for you. Part of weight loss is organization and preparation. Once you get into the swing of things and do a grocery shop for the food items you need, you are ready to get started.

A TYPICAL BALANCE DAY

- Start your day with a cup of warm water and freshly squeezed lemon juice 15 to 30 minutes before your first meal.
- Eat three meals and one to two snacks per day; do not skip the afternoon snack.
- If eating two snacks, one snack should consist of low-starch vegetables only.
- Eat three to four fat servings per day.
- Eat a minimum of three protein servings per day (1 protein unit per meal is suggested).
- Stop eating three hours before bedtime.
- Drink eight eight-ounce (250 mL) glasses of water per day.
- Work out three to five times per week.

If you follow the plan correctly, after three to five days you should no longer experience hunger or cravings. For best results, do not count calories or go hungry. Cutting too many calories from your diet will lower your metabolism, which is counterproductive to losing fat. If you are hungry or are working out quite a bit, opt for one of the free food choices or increase your protein intake by 1 to 2 ounces (30 to 60 g). Record all food items consumed in your Metabolism Boosting Food Journal (see page 271).

THE TYPICAL BALANCE PHASE DAY EXPLAINED

Behind the scenes of the BALANCE phase, there are specific reasons for each and every step. I am a firm believer that the more you understand the science and reasoning of the program, the better and longer lasting your results will be. By understanding the *why* of each step, the mystery will be taken out of weight loss. The information

"Free" foods

- starch-free vegetables (see page 145)
- vegetable or chicken broth, preferably low-sodium
- herbal teas and water
- herbs and spices

Limited foods

- 1 cup (250 mL) coffee or black tea per day
- 1 fibre-rich fruit per day
- 1/4 cup (60 mL) legumes per day
- 1 oz (30 g) goat's cheese or low-fat cheese per day

Food that will cut cravings

- 2 oz (60 g) additional protein
- homemade popsicles
- 1/2 cup (125 mL) unsweetened applesauce
- frozen grapes or mango chunks
- 2 chewable vitamin C tablets
- pickles (2 maximum) if craving salt
- 1 cup (250 mL) air-popped popcorn

You'll also find a list of foods specifically to cut salt cravings and sweet cravings on pages 164–165.

No-no foods

- aspartame
- alcohol
- sugar
- floury goods (bread, pasta, crackers, cookies, muffins, cakes, etc.)
- rice and potatoes

detailed in this section will forever be your "back pocket" tool for weight loss success. If life should throw you a curve ball and you feel your weight creeping back up, you will have the knowledge that will allow you to reel things back in and return to your goal weight.

START YOUR DAY WITH A CUP OF WARM WATER AND FRESHLY SQUEEZED LEMON JUICE

Traditional Chinese medicine has touted the benefits of lemon for centuries. High in antioxidants and vitamin C, lemon is a superstar fruit for myriad health complaints and can even be used for weight loss purposes. Lemon is a natural astringent and a "master cleanser" of the body. When consumed regularly, lemon juice can help to stimulate elimination in the digestive system and help purify the liver by removing by-products and waste matter. As we now know, digestion has a key role in a healthy weight loss program and daily elimination is essential. It is not unusual for someone to experience constipation in the early stages of any weight loss program. Regularly consuming warm water with freshly squeezed lemon will help to promote regular and healthy bowel movements.

Although lemons are acidic, they are alkalizing in the body, and the body thrives in an environment that is alkaline rather than acidic. Acid-forming foods (refined flours, sugars, alcohol, red meat, cheese) also tend to be the foods that promote weight gain, inflammation and sluggish bowels. See Appendix 6 for more information on acid and alkalizing foods.

Do not use bottled lemon juice as a substitute, as it can contain sulphites, which on rare occasions can cause allergic reactions. The benefits outlined above are with fresh lemons. Into 1 cup (250 mL) of warm water, squeeze the juice of 1/2 a fresh lemon. Drink 15 to 30 minutes before your first meal of the day, and feel free to drink more than a cup of lemon water per day or at night to curb cravings. If you do not like lemons, substitute limes.

EAT 3 MEALS AND 1 TO 2 SNACKS PER DAY; DO NOT SKIP THE AFTERNOON SNACK

To keep your blood sugars in balance, it is important to eat regularly and not skip any meals or snacks. For example, research is clear that people who skip breakfast tend to gain more weight in the long run. I suggest structuring your typical day as follows:

- Breakfast: 7 to 8 a.m.
- Morning snack: 10 a.m.—this snack is optional
- Lunch: noon to 1 p.m.
- Afternoon snack: 3 to 4 p.m.
- Dinner: 6 to 7 p.m.
- After dinner—free foods or drinks only

As you can see, eating every 3 to 4 hours from breakfast until dinnertime is ideal. If your timing is off from that listed above by an hour or so, do not panic; you are still on track. The key is to eat with enough regularity that you keep your blood sugars balanced. After dinner, stick to free foods only. Although you may skip the morning snack if you're not hungry, your afternoon snack is a must. Why? Because the body naturally has a blood sugar dip around 3 or 4 p.m. (a.k.a. the 3 p.m. slump, where fatigue and sugar cravings tend to pop up). If you eat a proper snack at this time, not only will you prevent the slump from occurring but you will also avoid a mini food binge before and after dinner. Snack options are outlined in the 7-Day BALANCE Meal Plan beginning on page 173.

IF EATING 2 SNACKS, 1 SNACK SHOULD CONSIST OF LOW-STARCH VEGETABLES ONLY

The starchy vegetables that are *not* allowed in this phase include beets, peas, acorn and butternut squash, parsnips, white potatoes, sweet potatoes, corn, rutabaga and plantain. Once you have completed the BALANCE phase, you can incorporate a limited amount of starchy vegetables into your diet.

Some diets suggest eliminating carrots because of their starch content, yet they are much lower in starch than the vegetables listed in the preceding paragraph. To this day, I have never had anyone at my weight loss clinic needing to lose weight because they have eaten too many carrots! Here are some ideal snack choices for your starch-free vegetable snack.

Recommended Starch-free Vegetable Snacks

- 1/2 cup (125 mL) sliced red bell pepper
- 1/2 sliced cucumber, lightly salted
- 1/2 cup (125 mL) tomato and cucumber salad, with balsamic vinaigrette if desired
- celery slices (as many as you like)
- lightly steamed broccoli or cauliflower with your choice of herbs or spices
- 10 baby carrots
- 5 to 10 cherry tomatoes
- 5 radishes
- 1/2 cup (125 mL) shredded cabbage with balsamic vinaigrette
- 1/2 cup (125 mL) green beans, lightly salted
- 1/2 cup (125 mL) sautéed zucchini
- 1/2 cup (125 mL) sautéed eggplant
- 1/2 cup (125 mL) hearts of palm
- 1 cup (250 mL) cooked rapini, spinach or kale, drizzled with olive oil and lightly salted
- 1 cup cooked bok choy with 1 tbsp (15 mL) sodium-light soy sauce
- 1/2 cup (125 mL) sautéed mushrooms and onions

If you are sautéing your vegetables in oil and eating them as a morning or afternoon snack, that is perfectly fine. As we'll discuss, the oil or fat you choose will count as one of your fat options. Keep in mind that you must consume a substantial amount of "good" fat in order to burn "bad" fat. Feel free to use any seasoning desired to spice up your vegetables. If choosing salt, use 1/4 teaspoon (1 mL) maximum.

EAT 3 TO 4 FUNCTIONAL FAT UNITS PER DAY

Functional fat units consist of the healthy fats, such as monounsaturated fats and omega-3 fats (discussed in Chapter 4). To boost metabolism and lose weight, you must consume a minimum of 3 and a maximum of 4 fat units daily. Fats are critical at this stage of weight loss, as they will fill you up; help to stabilize blood sugars, thereby reducing food cravings; support hormonal balance; keep energy up and support overall mood. I have seen people not lose weight effectively far too many times because they underconsumed healthy fats. Let's take a look at some recommended fat options.

Recommended Fat Options*

- 12 to 15 almonds
- 12 to 15 cashews
- 20 unsalted peanuts
- 25 to 30 unsalted pistachios
- 7 to 10 walnut halves
- 1/4 avocado
- 1 tbsp (15 mL) coconut oil
- 1 tbsp (15 mL) olive oil
- 1 tbsp (15 mL) sesame oil
- 1 tbsp (15 mL) butter
- 1 tbsp (15 mL) peanut, almond or cashew butter

- 1 tbsp (15 mL) ground flaxseed or flaxseed oil
- 1 tbsp (15 mL) hemp seeds
- 1 tbsp (15 mL) chia seeds
- 2 tbsp (30 mL) pumpkin seeds
- 2 tbsp (30 mL) sesame seeds
- 2 tbsp (30 mL) sunflower seeds
- 10 small green or black olives
- 1 tbsp (15 mL) oil-based salad dressing

*Each option = 1 fat unit

You'll notice that I've listed coconut oil as an option. Coconut oil has been shown to have numerous health benefits, including lowering cholesterol, being heart healthy and being nourishing for the hair and skin. It has even been shown to be beneficial for weight loss.

Unfortunately, coconut oil has gotten a bad rap because it is high in saturated fat. But there are different types of saturated fat—short-, medium- and long-chain. Unlike long-chain fatty acids, which must be emulsified by bile salts in the small intestine before they can be absorbed by the body, coconut oil is made up of short- and medium-chain fatty acids. These types of fats are immediately available to the body and can be digested and converted into quick energy. Thus, these types of fats do not contribute to obesity or weight gain when eaten in moderation because the body cannot store them. As well, coconut oil consists of 50% lauric acid, a fatty acid that has been shown to boost immune system function. If cooking on high heat, coconut oil, like sesame oil, is one of the most stable oils to cook with.

Here are some things you should know about fats.

- Many people tend to overdo it when it comes to eating nuts. If you do have an issue with portion control, count out the nuts and put them in individual bags or containers for snacking. (See Appendix 1, pages 282–285, for a list of the healthiest nuts to eat.)

- In addition to the recommended fat options given on the preceding list, I highly recommend taking a distilled fish oil supplement daily. Visit www.drjoey.com for suggested daily supplement intakes.
- Avoid frying with highly refined and processed oils such as canola (unless organic and expeller pressed), safflower, sunflower, soy or cottonseed oil. As a general rule, vegetable oils that are sold in plastic containers are not optimal for health.
- Some oils are healthier than others. See Appendix 4 for information on the healthiest fats to choose for cooking.
- Oil-based salad dressing used for topping vegetables is considered a fat unit (1 tbsp/15 mL = 1 fat unit).

EAT A MINIMUM OF 3 PROTEIN SERVINGS PER DAY

Of all the macronutrients, protein is often the missing link in weight loss. Although protein should not be the main source of fuel for your body (your body needs a sufficient amount of glucose from carbohydrates to run smoothly), it is a major player in stabilizing blood sugars and beginning the fat-burning process. Recall that protein stimulates glucagon, which leads to fat-burning. To stop the up-and-down swings of blood sugars that lead to weight gain, food binges, emotional eating patterns and fatigue, protein has to be consumed at each and every meal. I tell my clients to play the mental game of "name your protein" at breakfast, lunch and

> **EYEBALLING PORTION SIZES**
>
> A 3-ounce (90 g) cooked portion of a protein-rich food (e.g., fish, chicken, meat) is approximately the size of the palm of your hand (without fingers and thumb) or a deck of playing cards.

> **PORK—THE OTHER RED MEAT**
>
> Thanks to the very successful advertising campaign in the mid-1980s that positioned pork as "the other white meat," many people came to believe that pork is healthier than beef. However, the US Food and Drug Administration considers pork to be a red meat. Although pork is leaner than beef, it is significantly higher in saturated fat when compared with other lean protein sources. Lower fat protein sources are cold-water fish, poultry, eggs, egg whites, protein powders and soybeans.

dinner to ensure a high-quality protein source is present.

So, how much of a protein food should you consume per day? On average, in this phase, men should eat approximately 5 ounces (140 g) per meal; women should eat approximately 4 ounces (125 g) per meal. If you find you are hungry or are engaging in heavy physical exercise, you can increase your intake of protein-rich food by 1 to 2 ounces (30 to 60 g) per meal. The protein units listed in the table that follows contain anywhere from 6 to 40 grams of dietary protein per serving. Ideally, each meal should contain a minimum of 20 to 25 grams of dietary protein. This amount per meal is enough to make you feel satisfied, balance blood sugars and begin boosting your metabolism's engine. You can always combine protein sources (e.g., milk and protein powder in a smoothie) to increase your protein intake (see page 171 for how to make the perfect smoothie for weight loss). Red meat is not an ideal protein source because it tends to be high in saturated fat and can be inflammatory, but it can be consumed in very limited amounts (e.g., once every two weeks in the BALANCE phase).

Protein Content of Selected Foods

Food	Dietary protein (grams)
chicken, 4 oz (125 g)	28
fish, 4 oz (125 g)	28
extra-lean hamburger patty, 4 oz (125 g)	28
tuna, 6 oz (175 g)	40
cottage cheese, 1/2 cup (125 mL)	15
plain yogurt, 1/2 cup (125 mL)	5-8
Greek-style yogurt, 1/2 cup (125 mL)	10–12
skim milk, 1 cup (250 mL)	8
whey protein isolate powder, 1 scoop	15–20
tofu, 1/2 cup (125 mL)	20
1/2 cup (125 mL) edamame	11
legumes (including black beans, pinto beans and lentils), 1/2 cup (125 mL)	7–10
egg, 1 large	6

When choosing yogurt, avoid those with fruit bottoms or added granola, as they tend to be significantly higher in sugar than other types. Opt for Greek-style yogurt (available in most grocery stores), which is typically relatively low in sugar and calories. It's also thick, so it tends to fill you up while also satisfying your sugar craving. If you don't like plain yogurt, simply mix 1/4 cup (60 mL) plain yogurt with 1/4 cup (60 mL) of your favourite flavoured yogurt. This will give you your favourite flavour but with about half the sugar. Having said that, plain yogurt (Greek-style or other) is still the best choice.

STOP EATING 3 HOURS BEFORE BEDTIME

Over the years working with clients to boost nutrition and achieve weight loss, I have continually drawn on the practices of Ayurvedic medicine, a form of Indian traditional medicine that is more than 5,000 years old. Its principles, though not routinely spoken of in the allopathic medical model that we follow in North America, have benefited my clients enormously. One principle of Ayurvedic medicine is that, as the sun goes down, so does our metabolic capacity. In fact, Ayurveda practitioners believe that our metabolic strength is at its peak from noon to 2 p.m. (i.e., lunchtime). I have continually seen the beneficial weight loss and health effects of eating a lighter dinner in the evening. By doing so, you will wake up in the morning with more energy and a flatter stomach, and will quickly notice the pounds on the scale starting to drop.

JUST 1/2 CUP (125 ML) SHELLED EDAMAME (SOYBEANS) CONTAINS:

- 120 calories
- 4 grams fibre
- 3 grams fat
- 0.5 grams monounsaturated fat
- 11 grams protein
- 9 grams carbohydrate

For many weight loss seekers, putting an end to nighttime binging or emotional eating is often the hardest habit to break. What I can tell you for sure is that 9 times out of 10, eating late at night has nothing to do with real hunger (especially if you have consumed a proper dinner containing protein and fat). Nighttime eating often has emotional roots and can be linked to boredom, sadness, stress, or wanting a reward at the end of a tough day—or it may be a completely unconscious behaviour that has developed over many years.

To balance your blood sugars and lose your initial block of weight, there is no eating after dinner in the BALANCE phase with the exception of the free foods. In other words, if you are hungry after dinner, you may have starch-free vegetables (tomatoes, cucumbers, baby carrots, zucchini slices, bell peppers) or chicken broth to satisfy your need to eat. See also the recipe for Free Weight Loss Soup on page 181—a tasty option. Whenever I need to lose a few pounds, I always have this soup handy as a quick fill-me-up option. You can have 1 to 2 cups (250 to 500 mL) of this soup per day to fill up on as a free food.

DRINK EIGHT 8-OUNCE (250 ML) GLASSES OF WATER PER DAY

Not thirsty? That is the first sign that you are dehydrated and need to drink! Hydration is key to health and balanced energy, and an integral part of weight loss. In addition to promoting digestion and helping flush your system, drinking enough water ensures your liver does not become overtaxed—it's your liver that has to pick up the slack from the kidneys if they are dehydrated and not working properly. When the liver puts in overtime because the kidneys are water-deprived, it cannot metabolize fat as efficiently as it can when the kidneys are functioning properly and sets the body up for excess fat storage.

The key to drinking water is not to drink too much at once. Doing so is neither healthy nor practical. To incorporate this new routine into your life, simply pick 4 times per day to drink a glass of water, and sip the rest—the other 4 glasses—throughout the day. Keeping a water bottle on your desk or in your car will help make this new habit stick. To reduce our carbon footprint and for health reasons, it is best to avoid drinking water from a plastic bottle. Invest in a glass or stainless steel one.

I also recommend flat rather than carbonated drinks such as seltzer or soda water. Carbonated beverages can cause bloating due to the release of the carbon dioxide trapped in the bubbles. This contributes to gas in the stomach and can slow its emptying. Club soda often

HEALTH BENEFITS OF DRINKING WATER

- increased fat loss
- faster metabolism
- increased energy
- decreased joint pain
- regulated appetite
- reduced blood pressure
- regular bowel movements
- clearer skin

contains sodium bicarbonate, sodium phosphate or sodium citrate, all of which contribute to the 75 grams of sodium in an 8 ounce (250 mL) glass. Drinking carbonated beverages (even the sugar-free ones) can contribute to dehydration in the body. It is estimated that a glass of club soda is equal to the loss of a glass of water in the body. I have seen several clients follow the diet plan perfectly yet not lose a pound for a week or two because they were drinking so many carbonated beverages. As soon as the carbonated water was eliminated from the diet, their weight started to drop once again. Clearly, drinking plain water is the best option, but if you must choose the lesser of two evils, opt for sodium-free seltzer or sodium-free club soda.

By following this drinking guideline, you will quickly work your way up to eight 8-ounce (250 mL) glasses of water per day. Herbal teas can count as part of your water intake as well.

When drinking water, there are a few things you can do to take it up a notch for weight loss and health benefits. I highly recommend adding chlorophyll or a green powder to your water once daily; both support adrenal health. I also recommend keeping a jug of Weight Loss Water (page 154) handy. It is tasty and hydrating, and helps curb any and all sweet tooths.

WORK OUT 3 TO 5 TIMES PER WEEK

As a working mother of two little kids, I have found that for now, my days of hitting the gym for long workouts are over. Even so,

Weight Loss Water

8 1/2 cups (2.125 L) water
1 tsp (5 mL) grated ginger
1 medium cucumber, sliced
1 medium lemon or lime, sliced
10 spearmint leaves

Combine all ingredients and let stand in fridge overnight. Drink throughout the day.

my goal is to keep in great shape so I have the energy and mental clarity for all of life's demands. After researching the most effective way to maximize my workouts in the shortest amount of time, I discovered that high-intensity workouts (a.k.a. "HI" workouts) offer the greatest results. After recommending this approach to my weight loss clients (whether it was for toning, to break a plateau or to boost their metabolism), the results were clear: short, high-intensity workouts are the way to go.

Of course, engaging in regular physical activity is key to keeping your metabolic engine running at full throttle, thereby maximizing weight loss results. However, many people feel overwhelmed and even intimidated at the thought of changing their diet *and* starting a new exercise routine at the same time. In terms of exercise, the key to success is regularity and intensity, not time put in. In other words, regular, short workouts of 15 to 20 minutes at high intensities of strength (e.g., using heavy weights) and 20 to 30 minutes of cardiovascular activity (e.g., brisk walking, light jogging) will keep your metabolism running at its highest potential.

Even if you work out for shorter periods, fitting exercise into the day can often be the most difficult element of all. I would love to tell you it just magically happens, but it does not. In order to build exercise into your life, you have to plan for it. Consider these suggestions for making your life a little easier and to get you moving:

- If you lift weights at home, increase the weight and lift slowly. In other words, if you are doing bicep curls and can easily lift 10 pounds, the amount of muscle you will build and the challenge to your metabolism is not that great. To challenge your metabolism and muscle-building potential a little more, pick up a heavier weight (say, 15 pounds) and lift, going through the range of motion as slowly as you possibly can. Sounds easy? It actually is somewhat challenging at first. Although the time you put in doing this exercise is less, the intensity is greater because of the slower pace and increase in weight (you should be able to feel a slight burn). Fewer repetitions + slower pace + heavier weights = metabolic boosting!
- Invest in a piece of home equipment such as an elliptical or treadmill. Cardiovascular machines can now be purchased at greatly reduced prices on the Internet or at warehouse sales. There is nothing like having the convenience of working out at home. It is simple, accessible and a terrific option to turn to in the winter months. If you have a piece of equipment you have not used in a while, dust it off. If watching TV while on your treadmill or bike or listening to an iPod works for you, go for it!
- Find a buddy and power walk. Whether it is a neighbour, a friend or your spouse, a walking buddy will help motivate you to wake up half an hour early and get out there to walk briskly for 20 minutes. If you live in an area that has harsh winters, consider investing in some good gear that can allow you to walk outside comfortably.
- Practise yoga postures a minimum of 2 times per week. As a dedicated yoga student for the past 22 years, I can tell you that yoga is a life changer at both a physical and spiritual level. Outlining the practice of yoga is, of course, beyond the scope of this book, but I do encourage you to begin. Simply doing yogic sun salutations (a series of 12 postures performed in one single, graceful flow) will increase

both your strength and flexibility. In addition, yoga greatly reduces anxiety and stress, so practicing it will reduce your cortisol levels and help with weight loss and overall health. Starting your day off with 2 to 3 rounds of sun salutations will also affect the mood and pace of your entire day. For a visual of the sun salutations, visit http://www.yogasite.com/sunsalute.htm.

- Practice the Metabolism Boosting TV workout. The TV workout consists of squats, push-ups and sit-ups. While it's not necessary to do these techniques in front of the TV, watching TV is the perfect time to fit in a little muscle toning. In fact, you can easily address a wide variety of muscle groups in under 10 minutes simply by following the three "perfect" techniques that I'll outline in a moment.

The more weight you lose, the more you will need to tone by lifting weights and doing sit-ups, push-ups and cardiovascular exercise. This will help to ensure your muscles are more defined and strong. Be sure to consult a health care professional before engaging in any new exercise program.

The Metabolism Boosting TV Workout

The perfect squat

Squats are known as the "king" of all exercises, as they target the glutes, quadriceps and hamstrings. In short, if you want a tight tush, this is the exercise! Simple to do, squats can be done in the comfort of your home, in a gym or at the park. To do the "perfect" squat, I recommend beginning without weights.

Start by standing with your feet a little more than shoulder-width apart, to provide a sturdy base. Keeping your back as straight as possible (do not lean too far forward or too far back), lower yourself into a squat position. Try to imagine that you are sitting down on a chair. When moving into a squat position, your buttocks will lower toward the floor while your knees remain in line over your toes.

Contracting your abdominal muscles, lower yourself down as far as you can, aiming to bring your thighs parallel with the floor, then straighten your knees to lift yourself back up to the original standing position.

Once you feel comfortable with squats, proceed to walking squats (being careful not to sink into your knees) and squats holding light weights (5 to 7 lb/2.2 to 3.15 kg) by your sides.

When lifting weights, lift slowly and "put your mind in the muscle." In other words, focus on the muscle you are targeting by flexing up and expanding down, as in a bicep curl. Simply focusing on the tension and range of motion of the muscle you are engaging will produce greater results.

The perfect push-up

Push-ups are another incredibly effective way of muscle training your chest, shoulders and triceps. They can also be done in the comfort of your home, in a gym or at the park.

Start by kneeling on all fours, your hands slightly wider than your shoulders. Keeping your chin tucked in so your neck is aligned, contract your abdominal muscles and extend your legs out behind you in a plank position. The slower the motion the better, so count slowly to 10 while pushing up and then again while going down. As you lower yourself toward the floor, inhale slowly, allowing your elbows to bend outward away from your body until your chin is about 1 inch (2.5 cm) from the ground. Pause for 1 to 2 seconds before pushing back up slowly.

If you are new to push-ups, feel free to do a modified version where your knees are bent and resting on the floor or a mat, rather than being straight.

The perfect sit-up

Sit-ups are an integral part of any exercise routine and, for optimal abdominal results, should be done 6 times per week. Remember, this does not have to take a lot of your time. However, the repetition is necessary in order to see the definition and flattening you're looking for.

The perfect sit-up is quite easy. Simply lie on your back on a padded surface with your knees bent at 90 degrees and your feet flat on the floor. If you are a beginner, place your hands at your sides; for a more advanced position, move your hands closer to your head or cross them over your chest. To avoid a neck injury, never interlace your fingers behind your head or pull up on your head while executing sit-ups.

To start, lift yourself up slowly toward your knees as you exhale, pulling your navel toward your spine. When your upper torso is raised about 6 to 12 inches (15 to 30 cm) from the floor, pause and squeeze for a count of 5, tensing your core muscles. Lower yourself back down toward the floor as you inhale, stopping when you are lightly touching the floor (keeping your abdominal muscles taut the entire time) but not in a resting position. Repeat the motion. Try to connect to and visualize your abdominal muscles through the range of motion so that they are constantly engaged.

YOUR PERFECT EXERCISE WEEK

- Weight lifting—slow lifting with heavier weights 2 to 3 times per week (15 to 20 minutes per session)
- Cardiovascular exercise—brisk walking, jogging, running or sprinting 3 to 5 times per week (20 to 30 minutes per session)
- Yoga—sun salutations in the morning and light stretching 5 times per week (10 to 15 minutes per session)
- Metabolism Boosting TV Workout—squats, push-ups and sit-ups 3 to 5 times per week (10 minutes per session)

LIMITED FOODS

Certain foods and beverages are allowed in the BALANCE phase but must be consumed in limited quantities.

1 cup (250 mL) coffee or black tea per day

Whenever I do a lecture, I always say to the audience, "Put your hand up if you are a coffee drinker." Without fail, 80 to 90% of participants' hands go up. I too enjoy my one daily cup of java, but as with anything, moderation is key.

Drinking 1 cup (250 mL) coffee or black tea per day is the maximum amount you should be consuming in the BALANCE phase. As you know, in this phase it is necessary to start flushing the system of toxic waste and to begin balancing blood sugars. Caffeinated beverages such as coffee or tea can upset blood sugar balance and, if consumed in excess, can contribute to a state of dehydration and constipation, which will compromise your digestive health and weight loss results.

If you like flavouring in your coffee or tea, opt for skim milk with raw cane sugar, agave syrup or honey—1 teaspoon (5 mL) maximum. For weight loss purposes and health benefits, switch to green tea after enjoying your one coffee or black tea. In addition to lowering cholesterol and easing arthritic pain, 3 cups (750 mL) green tea per day helps to burn fat and boost metabolism. The active component in green tea, known as EGCG, appears to be responsible for the beneficial effect on weight loss. In addition, green tea secretes an amino acid called L-theanine, which creates a feeling of alertness yet calm. In fact, green tea can be the ideal replacement for coffee and a pick-me-up when experiencing the 3 p.m. slump. If drinking green tea makes you nauseous or does not appeal to you, try it in supplement form.

Here are some other natural coffee substitutes:

- ***Chai tea***—generally made with a base of black tea, with mixed spices such as ginger, cinnamon, cardamom, nutmeg and cloves; contains a small amount of caffeine.
- ***Roasted dandelion root tea***—has a roasted flavour, with a little bitterness. Good for detoxifying the liver.
- ***Rooibos tea***—from South Africa, also known as redbush tea. Like black tea, it is good with milk, but it's caffeine-free and full of antioxidants.
- ***Teeccino***—the number one coffee alternative in the U.S. This herbal "coffee" is perfect for anybody addicted to caffeine. It offers a great taste and none of the harmful side effects of coffee.
- ***Yerba maté***—caffeine-free tea with a stimulant effect and antioxidants.
- ***Matcha***—Japanese powdered green tea, very rich in antioxidants, fibre and chlorophyll. An energy booster!

1 fibre-rich fruit per day

One of my dearest weight loss clients was thrilled to hear she could eat fruit on the Metabolism Boosting Diet and still lose weight. The previous weight loss program she had been on had eliminated all fruits from her diet, the reasoning being that the sugars would hinder results. In truth, the right type of fruit ("nature's candy") will not bump around blood sugar levels or interfere with successful weight loss results. In fact, certain fruits are great go-tos to get you over your initial sugar hump. In the BALANCE phase, you are allowed 1 fibre-rich fruit option per day. When you move into the BOOST! phase, you will be allowed more fruit options. Your 1 fruit serving per day may be one of the following:

- 1 apple
- 1/2 banana
- 1/2 cup (125 mL) berries

- 1/2 cup (125 mL) cantaloupe or honeydew chunks
- 1/2 cup (125 mL) cherries
- 3 clementines
- 1 grapefruit
- 1/2 cup (125 mL) grapes, either red or green
- 1/2 cup (125 mL) mango chunks, fresh or frozen
- 1 orange
- 1 peach
- 1 pear
- 1 plum
- 1 pomegranate

In this stage, no pineapple, watermelon, figs or dates, and no sugary dried fruit (such as raisins) or fruit juice, are permitted. Although these fruits do offer health benefits, the BALANCE phase is designed to balance blood sugars, and the sugar levels in these fruits is too high.

1/4 cup (60 mL) legumes per day

Legumes are an excellent low-GI, high-fibre option to fill you up. Simply toss into a salad or soup, use as a side dish or take with you as a grab-and-go snack. Options include lentils, chickpeas (garbanzo beans), kidney beans, navy beans and black beans. If using canned beans or lentils, rinse them thoroughly first to reduce the sodium level.

> Most legumes (black beans, pinto beans, lentils) contain about 7 to 10 grams of protein per 1/2 cup (125 mL) when cooked.

An alternative to the 1/4 cup (60 mL) of legumes is 2 tablespoons (30 mL) of hummus (you'll find tasty recipes for hummus on pages 229 and 255).

1 ounce (30 g) goat's cheese or low-fat cheese per day

Cheese does offer a good source of protein and calcium, but if eaten in excess it can hinder weight loss results. For example, regular cheddar cheese has about 9 grams of fat per ounce, 6 grams of which are saturated. If you are a cheese lover, all you have to do is change your relationship with cheese. Instead of using it as a main ingredient in your meal, utilize it as a flavouring agent or an accent—for example, use soft goat's cheese in an omelet or crumbled over a salad, include low-fat mozzarella in a wrap or eat a piece of low-fat organic cheese with an apple as a snack. Several popular cheeses are available with reduced fat, including cheddar, Monterey Jack, mozzarella, Swiss, Colby and Muenster. Lower-fat cheeses tend to be milder in flavour than their regular-fat counterparts and have a slight rubbery texture, but they can still be quite good in sandwiches and wraps. Reduced-fat cheeses have approximately 6 grams of fat per ounce, with 4 grams of that being saturated. My favourite cheese for weight loss and health purposes (and flavour) is soft goat's cheese, as it is easily digested and has fewer calories and fat in comparison with cow's milk cheese.

Note that cottage cheese and yogurt count as a protein and are not included in the limit of 1 ounce (30 g) of cheese per day on the plan. One ounce (30 g) of cheese is approximately the size of your thumb.

STOP YOUR CRAVINGS

In the early stages of the BALANCE phase, your cravings may temporarily increase before they go away completely. My own mother, who was on my plan (and has subsequently lost 30 pounds), called me on day 3 and said, "Okay honey, now what? I could literally eat the paint off the walls!"

Once you are past the first 3 to 5 days, you will notice your cravings are significantly reduced or even gone. If your cravings do intensify and the urge to eat at night feels overwhelming, it is completely normal, and I assure you, this feeling will quickly pass. All you have to do is have a "clean" 3 to 5 days at the beginning and you are through the hard part.

Remember, *cravings are not a sign that you are weak;* rather, they are a sign that your blood sugars need balancing. Do not attempt to fight out your cravings—it never works and often results in food binging. By following the plan outlined in this chapter, you will crave no more. You may eat naturally sweet food, but you do not "need" it.

Let's look at the food options that you can turn to in order to satisfy your cravings.

- **2 ounces (60 g) additional protein**
  This is on top of your 3 protein units per day. Protein options to kill a craving are 1 hard-boiled egg, 2 slices of nitrate-free turkey or chicken, or a 100-gram container of plain yogurt.
- **Homemade popsicles**
  If you feel like a sweet, simply eat a homemade popsicle. Blend water with frozen berries, pour into a popsicle mould and freeze. Another option is to make an extra amount of your favourite protein-powder smoothie (see page 171 for simple smoothie steps, and Chapters 7 and 8 for recipes) and freeze it in a popsicle mould for a treat.
- **1/2 cup (125 mL) unsweetened applesauce**
  Low on the glycemic index and low in calories, unsweetened applesauce can cure any sweet craving.
- **Frozen grapes or mango chunks**
  Keeping a supply of frozen fruits available to grab in the first week of the program is enormously helpful in shutting down the craving for sweets. The frozen element helps because the fruit remains in your mouth longer. This small amount of frozen fruit does not count as your 1 fibre-rich fruit per day.

- **2 chewable vitamin C tablets**

  Vitamin C can help to satisfy your craving and "click off" the urge to overindulge. Chewable vitamin C can be purchased at most health food stores and pharmacies.
- **Pickles**

  Many people question why pickles may be used for cravings, since they are high in sodium. The reason is that no one binges on pickles! After one or two, you've had enough. One of the main goals of the foods you can turn to for help curbing cravings and emotional eating is that they "stop you in your tracks" and snap you back to awareness eating. If eating a pickle or two satisfies the urge to eat at night—no damage done.
- **1 cup (250 mL) air-popped popcorn**

  Just 1 cup (250 mL) of air-popped popcorn is filling yet it contains only 30 calories and a mere 6 grams of carbohydrates. Do not eat microwave popcorn. Air poppers can be purchased at most kitchen stores for under $20.

Salt cravings

If you are craving salt, try:

- cucumber pieces, lightly salted
- 1/4 avocado with a dash of sea salt
- 1/2 handful of lightly salted soy nuts
- Crispy Kale Chips (page 253)
- celery pieces, lightly salted

Sweet cravings

If you are craving sweets, try:

- sweet non-black teas—chocolate- or caramel-flavoured herbal teas, iced green teas, herbal and sweet fruit teas

- sweet vegetables like baby carrots, red bell peppers and sweet cherry tomatoes
- a sliced green apple or a glass of water with freshly-squeezed lemon

NO-NO FOODS

Certain foods are not allowed in the BALANCE phase. Why not? Because they either promote hunger, destabilize blood sugar levels or create the perfect environment for cravings to creep back in. The no-no foods are outlined here:

Aspartame

Research has shown that aspartame promotes fat storage and increased body mass index. It is not unusual for me to meet a client with forty pounds to lose who drinks 4 to 5 diet sodas per day!

Alcohol

You will see that a certain amount of alcohol is allowed in the next phase of weight loss. However, in the BALANCE phase, we are going to set the stage for metabolic boosting blood sugar control and by eliminating alcohol for 5, 10 or 15 days.

IS SEA SALT HEALTHIER THAN TABLE SALT?

Sea salt is derived from evaporated ocean water and goes through very little processing. Table salt comes from underground mines and is put through a chemical treatment process and is then typically fortified with iodine. White table salt is finely ground and bright white, whereas natural sea salt is grey because of its trace amounts of iron, calcium, zinc and iodine, which are typically lost in the refining of table salt. This does give sea salt a slight health edge, making it the preferred salt to use.

Regardless of which type of salt you use, I recommend keeping your sodium intake to between 1,300 milligrams and 2,400 milligrams per day. If you have high blood pressure, it is optimal to stay at the lower end. Bear in mind that 1 teaspoon (5 mL) salt contains 2,300 milligrams of sodium.

Sugar

Added white sugar, found in a variety of food products, will ring that insulin bell in your body, promoting fat storage, energy fluctuations and intense cravings for more. Be a label reader and avoid it.

Floury goods

These include bread, pasta, crackers, cookies, muffins, cakes, rice and potatoes. The body has no idea if it is eating straight white sugar, a piece of white bread, a processed muffin, a bagel or a can of pop. To the body it is all the same and is processed as sugar, which tends to lead to the oversecretion of insulin and the promotion of fat storage. In short: avoid all white flours and sugar. This rule is a game changer when it comes to weight loss.

COMMON QUESTIONS IN THE BALANCE PHASE

Q: Why do I crave sweets?

A: You are cravings sweets because you have been bouncing around your blood sugars, likely by consuming too many sugary refined flours and sweets or because of stress-elevated cortisol. The goal of the BALANCE phase is to stabilize blood sugars and take a sugar holiday. You will find your cravings subside within a very short time—less than 1 week. Sugar cravings are often times the strongest cravings of all addictions. They are also a major hindrance when trying to boost your metabolism and lose weight. After completing the BALANCE phase you will be able to eat more naturally sweet foods, but you will not feel as though you need them for energy or to satisfy a craving.

Q: Do I have to count calories in this phase?

A: No, please do not count calories—simply follow the guidelines. Remember, it is important not to go hungry during this phase, as this can slow down your metabolism. If you do feel hungry and you have eaten all of the foods suggested for the day, opt for free food options. A motto I would recommend keeping in mind is: Eat until you are sated, not stuffed. In other words, try eating until you are comfortably full (approximately 80% full), rather than eating until your pants feel a little too tight.

Q: *I am constipated—what should I do?*

A: It is very common to initially be constipated when changing your diet in any way. Here are some tips to try to keep your bowels moving:

- Add 1 heaping tbsp (20 mL) ground flaxseed or ground chia, or 1 tbsp (15 mL) flaxseed oil, to your morning yogurt.
- Although grain is not recommended in this phase, if you have not had a bowel movement for 3 days or longer, add 1/4 cup (60 mL) bran cereal to your morning breakfast. All-Bran Buds or Bran Flakes will do the trick.
- Be sure to drink 6 to 8 (8 oz/250mL) glasses of water per day.
- Exercise—the motion of exercise (brisk walking or light running) can help to improve bowel motility.
- Supplement with probiotics ("friendly" bacteria) daily. Be sure to purchase a probiotic with a mixed strain and a minimum of 5 billion organisms per capsule. Take 3 capsules directly before bedtime.
- Supplement with a green powder to ensure your body is alkaline and to optimize digestion.
- Take a calcium-magnesium powder supplement to get the bowels moving. See www.drjoey.com for specific supplement recommendations.

Q: *Are legumes a protein or a carbohydrate?*

A: Although legumes contain protein, they contain more carbohydrates and are therefore classified as such. As outlined, in the

BALANCE phase, you are allowed 1/4 cup (60 mL) legumes per day. If, however, you are a vegan or a vegetarian and need to eat legumes as a protein source, you may increase the serving size to between 1/2 and 3/4 cup (125 and 175 mL) per day.

Q: I work out quite a bit. Should I increase my food intake?

A: If you are working out quite a bit, you may need an extra snack per day or an extra 1 or 2 ounces (30 or 60 g) of protein per meal. Feel free to add these if you are working out intensely.

Q: I work out first thing in the morning. Do I need to eat before my workout?

A: It depends. Some people need a little something before their workout to avoid feeling light-headed. If you're one of these people, have your 1 daily piece of fruit or a 100-gram container of plain yogurt—your allowable 2 ounces (60 g) of additional protein— at this time of day to get you through your workout.

Q: Do I need to eat organic fruits and vegetables?

A: I am a huge advocate of eating organic food; however, I also understand budgetary constraints. Luckily, organic produce is now in high demand, which is driving down the cost of eating organic considerably. If you cannot afford to buy everything organic, choose to at least buy those fruits and vegetables that are the most heavily sprayed with pesticides in conventional farming.

According to the Environmental Working Group (EWG), a US-based research and advocacy organization, consumers can reduce their pesticide exposure by 80% by avoiding the most contaminated fruits and vegetables. The EWG has labelled these fruits and vegetables "The Dirty Dozen"; they are listed here from most to least contaminated. To reduce your exposure to pesticides, try to buy organic varieties of these foods:

THE DIRTY DOZEN

1. peaches
2. apples
3. bell peppers
4. celery
5. nectarines
6. strawberries
7. cherries
8. kale
9. lettuce
10. grapes (imported)
11. carrots
12. pears

The EWG has also created a list of fruits and vegetables that are least likely to contain pesticide residue, even if they are not organically grown. Known as "The Clean 15," they're listed here from most to least clean:

THE CLEAN 15

1. onions
2. avocados
3. sweet corn
4. pineapples
5. mangos
6. asparagus
7. sweet peas
8. kiwi
9. cabbage
10. eggplants
11. papayas
12. watermelon
13. broccoli
14. tomatoes
15. sweet potatoes

When it comes to eggs, dairy, poultry and red meat, if your budget allows, organic is also best. Wild salmon is also recommended, since it has low toxicity.

Q: I really enjoy pasta. Are there any tasty alternatives?

A: Yes, there are at least a couple of tasty substitutes for pasta. Shirataki noodles are gelatinous translucent Japanese noodles. They are low carbohydrate and gluten-free. They consist mostly of a dietary fibre called glucomannan and contain very few calories. Although they do not have much flavour on their own, they absorb other ingredients well—try them with tomato or soy sauce. These noodles can be found in most grocery and health foods stores. One portion is 1/2 cup (125 mL).

Zucchini ribbons are another good option. Using a vegetable peeler, cut zucchini into ribbons, turning it as you go. Warm 1 tbsp (15 mL) olive oil in a saucepan over medium heat and sauté with 1 clove crushed garlic for a few seconds. Add 1/4 cup (60 mL) tomato sauce and 1 tbsp (15 mL) chopped fresh oregano and simmer for a few minutes. Add zucchini, stirring until soft. Season with salt and pepper. One portion is 1 cup (250 mL).

Q: I really enjoy smoothies. Can I drink them as a meal replacement for breakfast, lunch or dinner?

A: Yes, absolutely. Smoothies are a quick and easy nutrient-dense meal—plus they're delicious and filling. You'll find several smoothie recipes in Chapters 7 and 8. Or simply follow the easy steps that follow to create the perfect smoothie for weight loss.

FOLLOW THE GUIDELINES BUT DON'T GET STUCK IN THE DETAILS

Frequently, clients come into my office in a panic because they have eaten one too many fats that day or feel that they have had an extra ounce or two of protein. They are so determined to follow the program perfectly that they get stuck in the details. While I encourage you to follow the guidelines as strictly as possibly, if you have an extra little bit of protein or fat, maybe because you were hungry or you weren't paying attention to the serving size, all is not lost. In other words, you did not blow it—the body does not work that way. Try to relax into this program and know that it is actually not that difficult to follow. Keep in mind that you are shifting toward your

Creating the Perfect Smoothie

Step 1—You will need 1 cup (250 mL) liquid, such as rice or soy milk, unsweetened almond milk, skim cow's milk, goat's milk, juice or water. In the BALANCE phase, juice in smoothies is not permitted. You can also use plain yogurt for a thick, creamy base. Choose Greek-style yogurts, which tend to be thicker, higher in protein and lower in sugar than other types. In this case, I recommend using 1/2 cup (125 mL) liquid and 1/2 cup (125 mL) yogurt.

Step 2—Add 1 or 2 scoops of high-quality whey protein isolate powder. When selecting a protein powder, choose one that is free of artificial sweeteners (go to www.drjoey.com for recommendations).

Step 3—Add high antioxidant fruits or vegetables. Frozen mixed berries or mangos, 1/2 a banana or peaches will all add delicious sweetness. Or toss in spinach or green powder. Consider adding ground flaxseed or flaxseed oil for an extra boost of fibre and omega-3 fats (1 tbsp/15 mL).

Step 4—Toss in 1/2 a handful of crushed ice to thicken the mixture.

Step 5—Blend ingredients together on high until liquid is fully circulating for about 1 minute.

healthiest you, your best self and optimal health and wellness. That will not happen overnight. Although you will feel (and see) results quite quickly, if you should have an "off" snack or meal, just jump back on board. Be easy on yourself—you are going to do great!

RECIPES AND MEAL PLANS

In the following pages, you will find a 7-day meal plan for the BALANCE phase and some additional recipes. Keep in mind that unless you experience a bout of constipation and need some extra bran in the morning, this phase of weight loss is grain-free.

You do not have to follow the meal plan precisely; you can create your own meals according to your dietary likes and dislikes. The meal plan is simply an example of what a typical day might look like in the BALANCE phase. If you have another meal or snack that is consistent with the BALANCE phase and that you enjoy, go for it!

The recipes too are meant as meal ideas to provide you with easy options that can be eaten at work, at home and on the go. You do not need to prepare each and every recipe; they are merely suggestions, meals I have developed over the years of working with my weight loss clients.

If you are like me (and so many others), when losing weight you tend to eat the same thing over and over again. Many people find that by doing this they stay safe in the parameters of weight loss. And it's not a problem to eat this way—you don't need tons of food variety to be successful at any of the Metabolism Boosting Diet phases. The degree of variety in the program really depends on your tastes.

Remember, it is very important to food journal at this time. A sample Metabolism Boosting Food Journal can be found on page 271.

7-DAY BALANCE MEAL PLAN—PHASE 1

DAY 1

Upon rising: Warm water with juice of 1/2 fresh lemon

Breakfast: Chocolate Peanut Butter and Banana Dream Smoothie (page 176)

Morning snack: Veggie sticks or Free Weight Loss Soup (page 181)

Lunch: Mixed Greens with Marinated Tofu (page 179)

Afternoon snack: 1/2 cup (125 mL) Greek-style yogurt topped with 1/2 sliced banana

Dinner: Faux Pasta with Meat Sauce (page 188)

After dinner: Free foods if desired

DAY 2

Upon rising: Warm water with juice of 1/2 fresh lemon

Breakfast: 1 Apple Pancake (page 178)

Morning snack: Veggie sticks or Free Weight Loss Soup (page 181)

Lunch: Heart-Healthy Tuna Salad (page 186) served on lettuce of your choice

Afternoon snack: 1/2 cup (125 mL) edamame

Dinner: 2 Turkey Tacos (page 191)

After dinner: Free foods if desired

DAY 3

Upon rising: Warm water with juice of 1/2 fresh lemon

Breakfast: Antioxidant Berry Blast Smoothie (page 176)

Morning snack: Carrots and celery sticks or 1/4 cup (60 mL) chickpeas mixed with tomato sauce

Lunch: Chicken Lettuce Wrap (page 187)

Afternoon snack: 1/2 cup (125 mL) plain or Greek yogurt with slivered almonds

Dinner: Veggielicious Miso Soup (page 183) topped with 5 oz (150 g) cubed tofu

After dinner: Free foods if desired

DAY 4

Upon rising: Warm water with juice of 1/2 fresh lemon

Breakfast: Morning Parfait (page 177)

Morning snack: Sliced red bell pepper and cherry tomatoes

Lunch: Large mixed greens salad with Mighty Miso Dressing (page 184) topped with 3 to 5 oz (90 to 150 g) cooked salmon

Afternoon snack: 1 cup (250 mL) Crispy Kale Chips (page 253)

Dinner: 1 serving of Anytime Egg Bake (page 180) with large side salad (with dressing of your choice)

After dinner: Free foods if desired

DAY 5

Upon rising: Warm water with juice of 1/2 fresh lemon

Breakfast: Banana Sundae Breakfast (page 177)

Morning snack: Veggie sticks or Free Weight Loss Soup (page 181)

Lunch: Chicken Lettuce Wrap (page 187)

Afternoon snack: 2 tbsp (30 mL) hummus with veggies

Dinner: Herb Roasted Salmon (page 189) served with Cauliflower Mash (page 185) and steamed broccoli

After dinner: Free foods if desired

DAY 6

Upon rising: Warm water with juice of 1/2 fresh lemon

Breakfast: Chocolate Peanut Butter and Banana Dream Smoothie (page 176)

Morning snack: Baby carrots with 1/2 cucumber, lightly salted

Lunch: Quick Chicken Stir-Fry (page 186)
Afternoon snack: 10 raw almonds
Dinner: Free Weight Loss Soup (page 181) served with 4 oz (125 g) roasted chicken and 1 tbsp (15 mL) hummus
After dinner: free foods if desired

DAY 7

Upon rising: Warm water with juice of 1/2 fresh lemon
Breakfast: 1 serving of Anytime Egg Bake (page 180)
Morning snack: Carrot and celery sticks, broccoli spears
Lunch: Vegetable Lentil Soup (page 182) with large side salad
Afternoon snack: 1 large green apple with 10 raw almonds
Dinner: High-Protein Balsamic Chicken (page 193) served with a large mixed greens salad
After dinner: Free foods if desired

BALANCE PHASE RECIPES

Chocolate Peanut Butter and Banana Dream Smoothie

Chocolate lovers rejoice, this one's for you. If you have a nut allergy or do not like peanut butter, simply omit that ingredient. (*Serves 1*)

1/2 frozen banana
1 scoop chocolate whey protein isolate powder
1 tbsp (15 mL) natural peanut butter
1 tsp (5 mL) cocoa powder (optional)
1 cup (250 mL) unsweetened vanilla almond milk
Handful of crushed ice

Blend all ingredients together, pour into a glass and enjoy.

Per serving: 296 calories, 12.5 g total fat, 27 g carbohydrates, 22 g protein, 4.5 g fibre, 13 g sugars

Antioxidant Berry Blast Smoothie

If you prefer, don't use the avocado in this smoothie, though it adds some creaminess. (*Serves 1*)

1/2 cup (125 mL) fresh or frozen berries
1 scoop vanilla whey protein isolate powder
1/4 avocado
1 cup (250 mL) skim milk
Handful of crushed ice

Blend all ingredients together, pour into a glass and enjoy.

Per serving: 276 calories, 8 g total fat, 28 g carbohydrates, 26 g protein, 6 g fibre, 5 g sugars

Morning Parfait

This is the perfect breakfast to grab since it takes only two minutes to make. Customize this parfait with berries of your choice. (*Serves 1*)

1/2 cup (125 mL) 1% cottage cheese
1/2 cup (125 mL) fresh berries
12 raw almonds, sliced
1 tbsp (15 mL) ground flaxseed

Put cottage cheese in a bowl and top with berries, almonds and flaxseed.

Per serving: 261 calories, 13 g total fat, 20 g carbohydrates, 20 g protein, 6 g fibre, 9 g sugars

Banana Sundae Breakfast

This tasty breakfast option combines two of my favourite things: sweetness and crunch. Rich in protein and omega-3s, this meal is sure to be a regular on your morning roster. (*Serves 1*)

1/2 cup (125 mL) plain yogurt
1/2 scoop chocolate or vanilla whey protein isolate powder
1/2 banana, sliced
4 walnuts, chopped

Mix yogurt with protein powder. Top with banana slices and walnuts.

Per serving: 258 calories, 7 g total fat, 25 g carbohydrates, 24 g protein, 2 g fibre, 16 g sugars

Apple Pancakes

These flourless and naturally sweet pancakes are a great breakfast option and a hit for weight loss. They will definitely be your new favourite go-to pancakes. (*Serves 1*)

1 egg
1/4 cup (60 mL) egg whites
1 medium apple, peeled
1 tsp (5 mL) cinnamon
1 tsp (5 mL) butter or olive oil

In a medium-size bowl, whisk egg and egg whites with a fork. Set aside.

In another bowl, grate apple, using your hands to squeeze out the juice. Discard juice or save for another use. Add grated apple to egg mixture. Stir in cinnamon.

In a pan over medium heat, add butter. Pour apple-egg mixture into the pan. Cook for 3 to 4 minutes or until starting to brown. Flip the pancake over and cook on the second side until brown.

Per serving: 327 calories, 9 g total fat, 21.5 g carbohydrates, 19 g protein, 4.5 g fibre, 14 g sugars

Mixed Greens with Marinated Tofu

(*Serves 1*)

4 to 5 oz (125 to 150 g) tofu, sliced
1 tbsp (15 mL) low-sodium soy sauce
2 cups (500 mL) mixed greens
1/2 cup (125 mL) water-packed artichoke hearts, drained
1/2 cup (125 mL) cherry tomatoes
1 oz (30 g) soft goat's cheese
1 sweet onion, thinly sliced
Handful of chopped fresh basil

Marinate tofu in soy sauce for 5 to 10 minutes. Remove from marinade and lightly pan-fry over medium heat; allow to cool.

Combine ingredients and drizzle with 1 tbsp (15 mL) balsamic vinegar and 1 tbsp (15 mL) olive oil.

Per serving: 402 calories, 25 g total fat, 29 g carbohydrates, 24 g protein, 12 g fibre, 6 g sugars

Anytime Egg Bake

The egg bake is a tasty, high-protein, flourless option that will keep you sufficiently full. Feel free to experiment with the vegetables, adding a variety of your favourites to the bake. (*Serves 3*)

2 tbsp (30 mL) olive oil
1 medium red onion, finely chopped
1 clove garlic, minced
2 cups (500 mL) broccoli florets
1 cup (250 mL) thinly sliced mushrooms
6 large eggs
1/2 cup (125 mL) crumbled goat's feta cheese
Sea salt

Preheat oven to 350°F (180°C).

Heat olive oil in a large skillet over medium heat. Sauté onion for 8 to 10 minutes, until soft and translucent. Add garlic, broccoli and mushrooms to skillet and sauté for 8 to 10 minutes, until broccoli softens slightly (it does not need to be fully cooked, as it will continue to cook in the oven).

In a large bowl, combine eggs, cheese and salt to taste. Stir in the sautéed vegetables, then pour mixture into an oiled 9 × 12 inch (23 × 30 cm) pie plate.

Bake for 30 to 35 minutes, until browned around the edges and cooked through. Let cool for 15 minutes before serving.

Per serving: 331 calories, 24 g total fat, 9.5 g carbohydrates, 19 g protein, 2.5 g fibre, 0.5 g sugars

Free Weight Loss Soup

Enjoy this soup any time of day and eat as much as you want. You'll find this soup is a real lifesaver when hunger or cravings creep up after dinner. (*Serves 10*)

6 cups (1.5 L) low-sodium vegetable or chicken broth (homemade or low-sodium)
1 can (28 oz/796 mL) diced tomatoes
2 cups (500 mL) finely chopped cabbage
1 cup (250 mL) finely chopped zucchini
1 cup (250 mL) diced onions
1 cup (250 mL) diced carrots
1 tbsp (15 mL) dried oregano
1 tbsp (15 mL) low-sodium soy sauce
1 tbsp (15 mL) olive oil
2 tsp (10 mL) tomato paste
1 tsp (5 mL) balsamic vinegar

Place all ingredients in a soup pot and bring to a soft boil. Reduce heat to low and simmer for 30 minutes or until vegetables are tender.

Per serving: 60.5 calories, 1.5 g total fat, 9 g carbohydrates, 2 g protein, 2 g fibre, 5 g sugars

Vegetable Lentil Soup

This tasty and filling soup is the perfect option to pack for work or to eat for a fill-me-up-dinner. Looking for evaporated cane juice? Visit your local health food store and go to the aisle with natural sweeteners. Cane juice should be stored in a tightly sealed container in a cool, dry place. It will keep indefinitely. (*Serves 8*)

1 cup (250 mL) dried green lentils
8 cups (2 L) vegetable broth
1 tbsp (15 mL) unsalted butter
1 cup (250 mL) diced zucchini
1/2 cup (125 mL) diced red bell pepper
1/2 cup (125 mL) chopped leeks
2 tsp (10 mL) sea salt
1 tsp (5 mL) evaporated cane juice
1/2 tsp (2 mL) black pepper
1/4 tsp (1 mL) white distilled vinegar
3 tbsp (50 mL) chopped fresh parsley

In a soup pot over medium heat, cook lentils in vegetable stock for 15 to 20 minutes or until lentils are soft.

In a large sauté pan over medium heat, sauté zucchini, bell pepper and leeks in butter for 5 to 7 minutes, until vegetables begin to soften. Add vegetables to stock and simmer for 10 minutes. Stir in salt, cane juice, pepper and vinegar.

Cool soup slightly, then transfer to a blender. Purée until smooth. Stir in parsley and serve.

Per serving: 100 calories, 2 g total fat, 15 g carbohydrates, 6 g protein, 8 g fibre, 2 g sugars

Veggielicious Miso Soup

Miso lovers, this one is for you! This filling soup is very low in calories but will still ensure you do not experience any hunger pangs while in the BALANCE phase. Miso can be found in the refrigerated section of most health food stores. In general, the darker the miso, the stronger the flavour. (*Serves 2*)

1 1/2 cups (375 mL) vegetable broth (homemade or low-sodium)
1/2 cup (125 mL) veggies of your choice (e.g., grated carrots and cabbage)
2 shiitake mushrooms, diced
2 green onions, chopped
1 tbsp (15 mL) high-quality organic miso
1 tsp (5 mL) sesame oil

In a soup pot, bring broth to a soft boil. Reduce heat to a simmer. Add veggies, including mushrooms and onions, to broth and simmer for about 5 minutes, until soft.

Remove soup from heat. Add miso and sesame oil. Stir well until miso is dissolved.

Per serving: 165 calories, 5 g total fat, 25 g carbohydrates, 3 g protein, 4 g fibre, 7 g sugars

Mighty Miso Dressing

This dressing is perfect for tossing with a green salad. The sweet agave syrup used in this dressing is low on the glycemic index and big on taste. However, as with any sweetener, natural or not, moderation is key. Feel free to double or triple the recipe so that you will have it in the fridge for later. (*Makes 2 tbsp or 30 mL*)

1 tbsp (15 mL) olive oil
2 tsp (10 mL) balsamic vinegar
1/2 tsp (2 mL) miso
1/2 tsp (2 mL) agave syrup
1/2 clove garlic, minced

Combine all ingredients.

Per serving: 75 calories, 6.5 g total fat, 1 g carbohydrates, .5 g protein, 0 g fibre, 2.5 g sugars

Cauliflower Mash

Looking for the perfect side dish to enjoy at lunch or dinner? This low-calorie and low-glycemic-index option is just as tasty and creamy as regular mashed potatoes. (*Serves 4*)

1 head cauliflower, broken or cut into pieces
1/4 onion
1 clove garlic, minced
1 tbsp (15 mL) butter
1 tbsp (15 mL) olive oil
Sea salt and freshly ground black pepper

Steam cauliflower, onion and garlic for about 10 minutes, or until cauliflower is tender but not mushy. Allow to cool for a couple of minutes.

Place cauliflower, onion, garlic, butter and olive oil in a food processor. Add salt and pepper to taste. Process until smooth and creamy.

Per serving (1 tbsp): 87 calories, 3 g total fat, 0.5 g carbohydrates, 0 g protein, 0 g fibre, 1 g sugars

Heart-Healthy Tuna Salad

Instead of using mayonnaise in your tuna salad, why not throw in heart-healthy mashed avocado? The healthy monounsaturated fat found in avocados will help you lose weight. (*Serves 2*)

1 can (6 1/2 oz/184 g) light tuna packed in water
1/2 fresh avocado, mashed
Juice of 1/2 a lemon
Large handful of fresh herbs of your choice
Chopped onion, celery or bell pepper (optional)
Dash of hot sauce (optional)

Mix ingredients together in a medium-size bowl. Enjoy on a piece of Romaine lettuce or Belgium endive or top on a salad.

Per serving: 180 calories, 7 g total fat, 7 g carbohydrates, 22 g protein, 3.5 g fibre, 0.5 g sugars

Quick Chicken Stir-Fry

(*Serves 1*)

4 oz (125 g) chicken strips
1 tbsp (15 mL) olive oil
1 cup (250 mL) assorted cut veggies (e.g., broccoli, carrots, onions, bok choy)
1 tsp (5 mL) tamari or low-sodium soy sauce

Stir-fry chicken for 3 minutes in olive oil, then add vegetables. Cook for 5 minutes. Stir in tamari and enjoy.

Per serving: 338 calories, 18 g total fat, 6 g carbohydrates, 38 g protein, 2 g fibre, 2 g sugars

Chicken Lettuce Wrap

(*Serves 1*)

4 oz (125 g) cooked chicken, cubed or sliced
2 to 3 large Romaine lettuce leaves
1/4 avocado
Salsa (store-bought or homemade)
Veggies of your choice (e.g., sliced cucumber or bell peppers)

Sprinkle chicken evenly down the centre of the lettuce leaves. Top with remaining ingredients and enjoy.

Per serving: 205 calories, 11 g total fat, 12 g carbohydrates, 20 g protein, 5 g fibre, 6 g sugars

Faux Pasta with Meat Sauce

Enjoy with a side salad. (*Serves 1*)

4 oz (125 g) ground, lean turkey
2 tsp (10 mL) olive oil
1/2 cup (125 mL) tomato sauce
2 to 3 mushrooms, sliced
1 zucchini

In a pan, sauté turkey in 1 tsp (5 mL) of the olive oil until no longer pink, breaking it up with a wooden spoon to avoid clumping. Add tomato sauce and mushrooms to turkey and simmer for 10 minutes.

Using a vegetable peeler, cut zucchini into ribbons, turning as you go, until you have approximately 1/2 cup (125 mL). In another pan, sauté zucchini noodles in the remaining 1 tsp (5 mL) olive oil until softened.

Place zucchini noodles on a plate and top with meat sauce.

Per serving: 287 calories, 16 g total fat, 12 g carbohydrates, 26 g protein, 2 g fibre, 9 g sugars

Herb-Roasted Salmon

Enjoy with a side salad or sautéed vegetable medley. (*Serves 6*)

1/3 cup (75 mL) cilantro
1/3 cup (75 mL) chopped dill
1/3 cup (75 mL) finely chopped green onions
1 tbsp (15 mL) olive oil
1 tbsp (15 mL) red wine vinegar
1 tbsp (15 mL) Dijon mustard
Sea salt
6 wild salmon fillets (approx. 4 oz/125 g each)

Preheat oven to 350°F (180°C).

In a small food processor, combine cilantro, dill, green onions, oil, vinegar and mustard.

Sprinkle fillets with a little salt and coat each side evenly with herb mixture. Arrange on a baking sheet.

Roast in oven until fish flakes easily when tested with the tip of a sharp knife, about 10 to 15 minutes, depending on thickness of fillets.

Per serving: 229 calories, 11 g total fat, 1 g carbohydrates, 22 g protein, 0 g fibre, 0 g sugars

Low-Carb Eggplant Bake

This satisfying dish will make you feel like you are eating a gourmet Italian meal—guilt free! Enjoy with a side salad for dinner.
(*Serves 4*)

1 large eggplant
2 tbsp (30 mL) olive oil
1 cup (250 mL) tomato sauce
1/2 cup (125 mL) soft goat's cheese
1/2 cup (125 mL) sliced mushrooms

Preheat oven to 375°F (190°C).

Cut eggplant into 1/4-inch- (5 mm) thick round slices. Pour 1 tbsp (15 mL) of the olive oil into non-stick medium-size pan, add eggplant and sauté over medium heat, 2 minutes per side.

Place eggplant in foil-lined medium-size casserole dish. Pour tomato sauce over top, then dot with goat's cheese. Bake for about 20 minutes or until brown and bubbly.

In a separate pan, sauté mushrooms in remaining 1 tbsp (15 mL) olive oil over medium heat for 4 to 6 minutes. Remove casserole from oven and top with sautéed mushrooms.

Per serving: 170 calories, 10 g total fat, 12 g carbohydrates, 10 g protein, 2 g fibre, 0 g sugars

Turkey Tacos

This is the perfect recipe if you enjoy the taste of tacos but can do without the carbohydrates from grains. You will find these tacos fill you up and are just as satisfying as those made with taco shells. (*Serves 4*)

1 tsp (5 mL) olive oil
1 lb (500 g) lean ground turkey
2 tbsp (30 mL) taco seasoning (see page 192)
1/4 cup (60 mL) water
8 whole Romaine lettuce leaves

Garnishes
1 tomato, chopped
1 avocado, sliced
1/2 onion, chopped
1 cup (250 mL) salsa (store-bought or homemade)
1/2 cup (125 mL) crumbled soft goat's cheese

Heat pan over medium heat. Add olive oil and turkey. Cook turkey until no longer pink, breaking it up with a wooden spoon to avoid clumping.

Add taco seasoning and water, stirring until well combined. Let simmer until sauce thickens, about 3 to 4 minutes.

Distribute the turkey mixture among lettuce leaves. Top with garnishes.

Per serving (2 tacos): 337 calories, 21 g total fat, 12 g carbohydrates, 28 g protein, 5 g fibre, 0 g sugars

Homemade Taco Seasoning

Use this seasoning for Turkey Tacos (previous page). (*Makes 1 cup or 250 mL*)

1/4 cup (60 mL) chili powder
2 tbsp (30 mL) ground cumin
2 tbsp (30 mL) onion powder
1 tbsp (15 mL) garlic powder
1 tbsp (15 mL) brown sugar
1 tbsp (15 mL) arrowroot
1 tbsp (15 mL) paprika
1 tbsp (15 mL) dried oregano
2 tsp (10 mL) sea salt

Combine ingredients and store in an airtight jar until ready to use.

High-Protein Balsamic Chicken

This high-protein chicken dish is a quick and easy dinner the entire family will enjoy. For those family members who are not in the BALANCE phase, simply serve theirs with brown rice on the side. This way, you won't be cooking two different dinners. (*Serves 1*)

1/2 cup (125 mL) balsamic vinegar
1/2 cup (125 mL) sliced mushrooms
1/2 cup (125 mL) sliced red and green bell peppers
Onion flakes
Sea salt and black pepper
5 oz (150 g) boneless chicken breast

Preheat oven to 350°F (180°C).

In a bowl, stir vinegar, mushrooms, bell peppers and onion flakes to taste. Add salt and pepper to taste. Pour mixture over chicken. Bake for 30 minutes or until chicken is cooked through.

Enjoy with a side salad, or 1 cup (250 mL) cooked broccoli or rapini.

Per serving: 311 calories, 11 g total fat, 4 g carbohydrates, 43 g protein, 1 g fibre, 2 g sugars

Shirataki Noodles with Edamame, Sun-Dried Tomatoes and Goat's Cheese

Shirataki noodles are found in most grocery and health food stores. they make the perfect low-calorie and low-carbohydrate alternative to pasta. (*Serves 4*)

1 pkg (8 oz/250 g) shirataki noodles
1 tbsp (15 mL) olive oil
1 cup (250 mL) dry-packed sun-dried tomatoes, thinly sliced
1/4 cup (60 mL) frozen shelled edamame, thawed
2 tsp (10 mL) minced garlic
1/4 tsp (1 mL) red pepper flakes (optional)
4 oz (125 g) soft goat's cheese, crumbled, plus more for topping
1/2 cup (125 mL) chopped fresh dill
Coarse salt and freshly ground black pepper

Remove noodles from package, rinse well and cook in boiling water for 2 to 3 minutes, then drain.

Heat a small skillet over medium heat. Add oil, noodles, sun-dried tomatoes, edamame, garlic and red pepper flakes. Cook, stirring occasionally, until fragrant, 1 to 2 minutes. Remove from heat.

Add goat's cheese, dill and salt and pepper to taste. Let stand approximately 5 minutes to thicken. Top with extra goat's cheese and serve.

Per serving (without extra topping): 180 calories, 11.5 g total fat, 6.5 g carbohydrates, 8 g protein, 2 g fibre, 1 g sugars

CHAPTER 8
PHASE 2: BOOST!

I think I can. I think I can. I know I can.
—From *The Little Engine That Could*

You did it! You successfully completed the initial BALANCE phase (which you followed for 5, 10 or 15 days depending on your score on the Metabolic ID Questionnaire in Chapter 6) and are now are ready to move on to the BOOST! phase. At this point, I'm sure you are wondering, "Okay, what changes in this phase?" As you will soon discover, in the BOOST! phase, you'll add in more food options that will both help fill you up and tempt your palate. Even so, the types and combinations of foods you will be eating are designed to maintain blood sugar control and to follow fat-burning and metabolic-boosting principles to ensure you reach your goal weight.

BENEFITS OF THE BOOST! PHASE

The benefits of this phase include continual loss of belly fat, ongoing weight loss, boosting of metabolism and improvement of energy, mood and digestive health. During this phase you will break the weight loss plateau and get all the way to your target weight. The BOOST! phase will also be when you begin to shift your patterns and relationship with food, finally putting an end to emotional habits, such as binge eating and nighttime eating.

LENGTH OF THE BOOST! PHASE

The length of the BOOST! phase will vary according to how much weight you have to lose. In this phase of the program, with exercise you will likely experience ongoing weight loss results of 2 to 4 pounds (1 to 2 kg) per week. Most likely, this will be the weight loss phase where you will remain the longest. You will move on to the next phase, MAINTAINANCE, once you hit your target weight in the BOOST! phase.

The objective of this stage is not rapid weight loss (e.g., 8 pounds every week). More often than not, rapid weight loss results in muscle wasting, poor digestive health and lack of energy. It is also not weight that tends to stay off long term. I constantly witness rapid weight loss resulting in rapid weight gain at some point down the line. Keep asking yourself that ever-important weight loss question, "Can I see myself following a version of this program in 5 years' time?" If not, then what is the point? As you will see, once you hit your goal weight, maintaining blood sugar control and hormonal balance to keep your weight off for life is a critical and permanent shift to long-term success. When in MAINTENANCE, you will certainly be able to eat more and indulge more often, but there are also fundamental, easy-to-implement principles that you must adhere to for lifelong weight loss success.

My most successful weight loss clients are those who are not in a race. In other words, these individuals have committed to losing the weight and getting healthy. If it takes them 4 months instead of 3, they are okay with that. As you will learn later on in the book, your weight loss momentum may not occur in a straight line. Most weeks you will lose between 2 to 4 pounds (1 to 2 kg) and will feel motivated and encouraged to continue. However, there likely will be occasional lacklustre weeks where you may lose only 1/2 pound or even no weight at all. Fear not: I will show you how to pick up your weight loss pace once again and make it to the finish line to hit your target goal weight. I also encourage you to continue working out 3 to 5 times per week. The dietary food plan outlined in these chapters along with the short, high-intensity workouts are critical when it comes to losing weight and keeping it off. At the end of this chapter, you will also find the 7-Day BOOST! Meal Plan, along with scrumptious and easy-to-make recipes.

THE BOOST! PHASE CHANGES EXPLAINED

In addition to keeping to the dietary structure outlined in Chapter 7, you'll need to implement additional changes in the BOOST! phase:

- Introduce 1 grain at breakfast or lunch
- Do not eat grain past 3 p.m.
- Feel free to add in 1 extra fruit option
- Enjoy 2 snacks per day
- Enjoy starchy vegetables 1 time per week maximum
- Enjoy 1 alcoholic beverage per week
- Use 1 free ticket per week

INTRODUCE 1 GRAIN AT BREAKFAST OR LUNCH

Yay! You get to add grain back into your diet. When eaten correctly and in moderation, grain—be it bread, rice, pasta, quinoa, whole-grain crackers, cereal or tortillas—can be a delicious part of your diet that can also help you to lose weight. While overconsumption of the wrong type of grain (white, refined and processed flour) leads to an increase in insulin and fat storage, the right type, filled with fibre and protein and lower on the glycemic index, promotes healthy digestion and can fill you up.

Recently, there have been some very popular diets that promote total elimination of grain from the diet in order for you to hit and remain at your target weight. If you do have a sensitivity to grain (e.g., are sensitive to wheat, have trouble digesting gluten), then a significant reduction is likely a good idea. (See "How do I know if I am sensitive to wheat?" in the Q&A section that follows.) But if you have no grain sensitivity or allergy, you're likely among those people who need a modest amount of daily whole grain to provide significant fuel and to satiate. I am a huge advocate of going organic with the grain options or selecting a grain that has undergone very little processing, such as sprouted grain or whole-grain rye bread.

In the BOOST! phase, the 1 grain option per day might be:

- 1 whole-grain tortilla (wrap)
- 2 pieces of whole-grain or spouted-grain bread (may be consumed at the same meal or divided between breakfast and lunch)
- 1/2 cup (125 mL) cooked brown rice or quinoa
- 6 to 10 whole-grain crackers
- 1/2 cup (125 mL) cooked whole-grain or spelt pasta
- 3/4 cup (175 mL) whole-grain, low-sugar cereal

See www.drjoey.com for bread and cereal recommendations.

Common questions about grains in the BOOST! phase

Q: Why sprouted-grain bread?

A: When a grain is sprouted, a portion of the starch content is predigested, which lowers the grain's GI value, making it ideal bread for weight loss. In addition, sprouted-grain bread provides more minerals and vitamins than regular bread and is generally made with unrefined and natural ingredients. Sprouted-grain breads are available in most grocery and health food stores. If you cannot find sprouted-grain bread, whole-grain bread or 100% whole-wheat bread is the next best thing.

> If you have had an issue with portion control in the past, do not opt for crackers, even if whole grain, as your grain option. It is far too easy to grab extra crackers when feeling blue, bored or tired. Opt instead for bread, a tortilla, quinoa or brown rice.

Q: What is quinoa?

A: Quinoa (pronounced "keen-wah") is actually not a grain but a seed. It has gained enormous popularity recently thanks to its high protein levels (it is a complete protein containing all nine essential amino acids) and because it is gluten-free, it is a perfect option for those who are gluten sensitive or celiac.

Before cooking quinoa, be sure to rinse the seeds well to remove their bitter, resin-like coating, called saponin. Cooked quinoa is excellent in casseroles, soups, stews and stir-fries, and also cold in salads. The seeds are prepared similar to rice and cook very quickly—in about 15 minutes. Simply boil 2 cups (500 mL) water for every 1 cup (250 mL) quinoa, put a tight-fitting lid on the pot and let simmer for 12 to 15 minutes or until the germ separates from the seed (it will look like a little curly tail on the kernel). Remove from heat and let stand for about 3 minutes, then fluff with a fork.

Q: How do I know if I am sensitive to wheat?

A: There are myriad symptoms of wheat sensitivity, such as inability to lose weight, digestive complaints (including gas, bloating and constipation), skin breakouts, fatigue, fogginess, joint pain, dry cough and headaches. If you do suspect you are having a reaction to wheat products, start to food journal for 1 to 2 weeks, documenting everything you eat that contains wheat. Wheat is found in white flour, whole-wheat flour, semolina, durum, triticale, couscous, tabbouleh, bran, modified food starch, gluten, bulgur, cake flour, pastry flour, graham, semolina, wheat bran, wheat germ and wheat starch. Most noodles and baked products also contain wheat.

After you have clearly identified where the wheat in your diet is, eliminate all wheat products for a 2-week period. Be strict, and keep notes in your food journal on how you feel and how the weight loss process is going. I have found that my clients who are sensitive to wheat have a weight loss *whoosh* once it is removed. In other words, the weight starts to just fall off. After avoiding wheat for 2 weeks, it is time to test and challenge your system with wheat products. For a 1- or 2-day period, introduce wheat back into your diet, closely monitoring how you feel and how your digestive system reacts. If you truly are sensitive to wheat, your symptoms or discomfort will return quickly and the needle on the weight scale will tend to go up.

Q: How do I know if I am sensitive to gluten?

A: Gluten sensitivity or intolerance is often confused with wheat sensitivity and can be difficult to diagnose without the help of a medical doctor. People with a gluten sensitivity or intolerance react to the proteins gliadin and glutenin that make up 80% of gluten.

Gluten is used to make baked goods more elastic and chewier. The shortlist of gluten-containing grains is wheat, barley, oats, spelt, kamut, rye and triticale. Grains that are given the green light for those who are gluten sensitive include basmati rice, brown rice, quinoa, amaranth, buckwheat (like quinoa, technically a seed but classified as a grain) and millet. Gluten sensitivity or intolerance is medically termed *celiac disease* or, more specifically, *celiac sprue.* Common symptoms include stomach cramping, nausea and vomiting, diarrhea, constipation, gas, acid reflux, fatigue, joint pain, infertility and ulcers.

> Did you know that grains such as barley, corn and rice generally have less than half the protein of quinoa? Quinoa is 12% to 18% protein. Four ounces (125 g) of quinoa per day (about 1/2 cup/125 mL) will provide a child's daily protein requirements.

Q: What if I am eating out and there is no suitable grain option available?

A: If you are dining out and there is no suitable grain option on the menu, simply drop the grain option for the day and stick to protein and vegetables. If you feel hungry, fill up on extra protein—a tuna salad, salmon with vegetables or chicken salad are all good choices.

Q: What is considered a low-sugar cereal?

A: Some cereals that are promoted as healthy still contain a significant amount of sugar. When looking for the sugar content of a cereal, check the Nutrition Facts table—the amount of sugar per serving will be listed. A passable cereal has less than 10 grams of sugar per serving. If you go double digits with your sugar intake, you have gone way too high. For example, if a serving size of

> Did you know that cooking pasta al dente (so it's firm when bitten) lowers its GI value and is a great trick for weight loss?

3/4 cup (175 mL) cereal contains 16 grams of sugar, that translates into 4 teaspoons (20 mL) of sugar (1 tsp/5 mL sugar equals 4 grams), which is quite a bit. You can also check the ingredient list to ensure that one of the first few ingredients listed is not sugar, since ingredients are listed from greatest to least amount used—watch for sugar, sucrose, glucose, fructose, cane sugar, dextrose, fruit juice concentrate, malt, molasses and honey.

Q: What about eating granola?

A: Although granola seems like it would be a healthy option, it is often high in sugar, fat and calories. If your granola seems fairly low in calories, check the label to see what the recommended portion size is—1/4 cup (60 mL) granola, for example, is not very much. Lower-fat versions of granola simply swap fat for sugar, which raises the GI value and contributes to blood sugar fluctuations and food cravings. Stick with a tiny amount of granola and use it just as a topping over yogurt.

DO NOT EAT GRAIN PAST 3 P.M.

For optimal weight loss results, do not eat grain past your afternoon snack. Your metabolism does not want to have a big, heavy meal—a plate of pasta, say—in the evening. Rather, it is best to lighten up from your 3 p.m. snack onward to boost metabolic function and energy and to burn abdominal fat. Like the old saying goes, eat breakfast like a king, lunch like a prince and dinner like a pauper. Unfortunately, in North America we tend to have a backward approach. We often skip breakfast, eat a high-GI lunch and enter the dinner hour feeling starving. By doing so, we are lining up the perfect scenario for a full and mindless food binge before dinner and for the rest of the evening. For optimal weight loss results, remember the words *supper is supplementary.* In a nutshell, dinner should be your lightest and smallest meal of the day. The figure that follows illustrates the ideal daily eating structure.

The Metabolism Boosting Ideal-Meal Pyramid

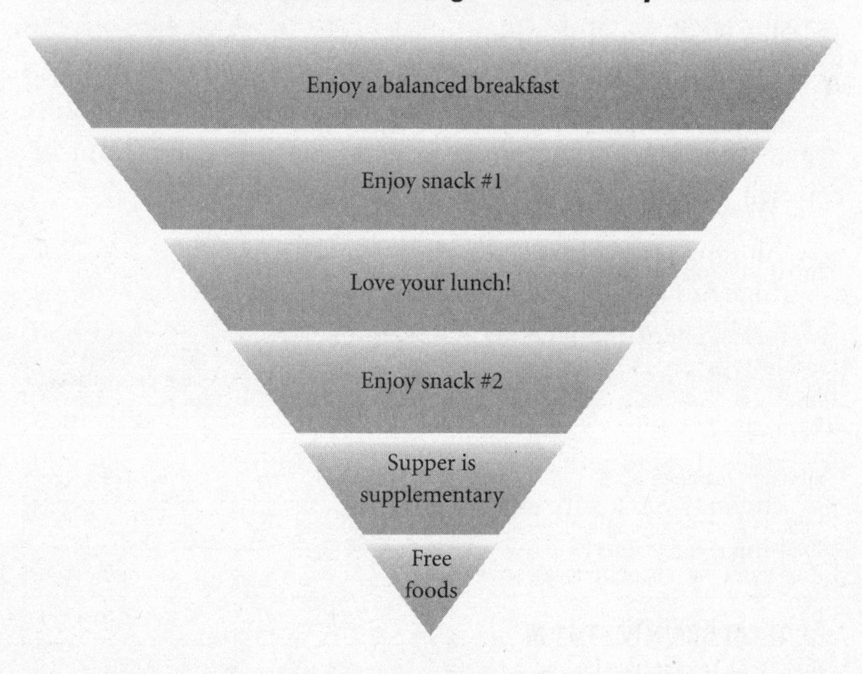

FEEL FREE TO ADD IN 1 EXTRA FRUIT OPTION

At this stage of weight loss, you may increase your fruit consumption to 2 servings per day. The fruits recommended are the same as those outlined in the BALANCE phase (see pages 160–161), with the addition of pineapple (1/2 cup/125 mL maximum) and watermelon (1/2 cup/125 mL or 1 Watermelon Popsicle, recipe page 239) if desired. It is best to avoid sugary dried fruit, including raisins, figs and dates, because of their high sugar content. Baked apples, or unsweetened, dried fruit like apple rings and apricots that have not been sugared may also be eaten as a fruit option (1 serving = 1 baked apple *or* 6 to 7 apricots *or* 10 pieces of dried apple).

When eating dried fruits, we tend to consume more calories than we would if we ate the same amount of fresh fruit. For example, 1/4 cup (60 mL) dried apricots contains approximately 75 calories and 17.4 grams of sugar. For that amount of calories, you could actually enjoy an entire cup of fresh apricots, which contains less sugar—14.3 grams. The chart below, which compares fresh versus dried apricots (the values of apricots being typical of those of other fruits), shows that dried fruits also tend to lose some of their nutrient richness.

Nutrient Comparison Chart

Nutrient	Fresh Apricots (per 1 cup/250 mL)	Dried Apricots (per 1 cup/250 mL)
Calories	74.0	313.0
Fibre (grams/calorie)	0.4	0.3
Vitamin A (international units/calorie)	40.3	15.0
Beta carotene (micrograms/calorie)	22.9	9.0
Vitamin C (grams/calorie)	2.0	0.0
Potassium (milligrams/calorie)	5.4	4.8

Source: http://www.whfoods.com/genpage.php?thame=george&dbid=170

Consider investing in a home dehydrator for making healthier dried fruit and vegetable options. However, fresh is still best—it is much easier to overdo it with dried apple pieces than with fresh apples.

ENJOY 2 SNACKS PER DAY

During Phase 1, the BALANCE phase, you were allowed to eat 2 snacks per day, but one of them had to be starch-free vegetables (e.g., baby carrots, celery sticks, cherry tomatoes). In Phase 2, the BOOST! phase, you can now enjoy 2 snacks per day from a variety of food choices (fruits, vegetables, nuts, seeds). Keep in mind that if you choose a protein bar or whole-grain granola bar as one of your snacks, it counts as your 1 grain per day.

Other snack option ideas include:

- carrot sticks with 2 tbsp (30 mL) hummus
- cucumber with 2 tbsp (30 mL) hummus
- celery sticks with 1 tbsp (15 mL) almond or peanut butter
- sweet bell peppers and 2 tbsp (30 mL) hummus or yogurt ranch dip
- 4 zucchini slices topped with 1 tsp (5 mL) pesto and 1 oz (30 g) low-fat cheese, thinly sliced
- 1/2 sliced green apple with 1 tbsp (15 mL) almond butter
- 1/2 cup (125 mL) unsweetened applesauce
- 1/2 cup (125 mL) watermelon and 1/2 cup (125 mL) roasted soy nuts
- 1/2 cup (125 mL) plain yogurt with 1/2 cup (125 mL) fresh berries
- 1/2 cup (125 mL) cottage cheese with 1/2 cup (125 mL) fresh berries
- 1/4 cup (60 mL) plain yogurt with 1 scoop chocolate whey protein isolate powder
- 1/4 cup (60 mL) plain yogurt with your favourite fresh herbs and lemon juice—serve with chopped veggies
- protein smoothie pops—freeze your favourite protein-powder smoothie in popsicle holders
- 1 hard boiled egg, lightly salted
- 1 to 2 cups (250 to 500 mL) Crispy Kale Chips (page 253)
- 1/2 cup (125 mL) edamame
- 1/2 cup (125 mL) mango chunks and 1 tbsp (15 mL) pumpkin seeds

- 2 small kiwis and 6 raw almonds
- 3 sliced apricots and 1 tbsp (15 mL) hemp seeds
- 10 raw almonds or walnuts
- 10 tamari-roasted almonds
- 30 pistachios
- 5 whole-grain crackers topped with 1 tsp (5 mL) tomato sauce and 1 oz (30 g) low-fat cheese—for mini-pizzas, melt the cheese

ENJOY STARCHY VEGETABLES 1 TIME PER WEEK MAXIMUM

To fill up and add variety to your diet, you may add in 1 starchy vegetable per week if desired (not mandatory), such as one of the following:

- beets (1/2 cup/125 mL)
- corn (1/2 cup/125 mL)
- squash (1/2 cup/125 mL)
- yam or sweet potato (1 small, the size of an average baseball)

White potatoes are not permitted.

ENJOY 1 ALCOHOLIC BEVERAGE PER WEEK

For some, giving up alcohol altogether is no big deal and it is simply not missed. If you are one of those individuals, you do not need to introduce alcohol to your diet at this point. However, if you do enjoy a glass of red wine or other alcoholic beverage in the evening, feel free to enjoy 1 per week. If consuming only 1 drink per week sounds far

A STANDARD DRINK IS

- 12 ounces (355 mL) of regular beer
- 5 ounces (150 mL) of wine
- 1 1/2 ounces (45 mL) or a "shot" of spirits

too little an amount for you to stick to, do not fear. As you will soon learn, you also have 1 free ticket per week that you can cash in on whatever you like. You may decide to use that ticket for an alcoholic drink at dinner once per week.

As you now know, part of your weight loss success will be attributable to balanced blood sugar levels and a reduction of the fat-storing hormone insulin. The problem with alcohol is that the body treats it like a sugar, which can trigger fat storage. Thus, any more than 2 drinks per week may hinder your weight loss.

Common questions about alcohol in the BOOST! phase

Q: What do I do if I want more than 2 drinks per week?

A: In phase 2, the BOOST! phase, you're allowed 2 drinks per week: 1 per week is allowed, plus you can cash in your free ticket for an extra alcoholic beverage if you like. If you find this overly restrictive for your lifestyle and want to consume more, then amends will have to be made in other areas of your dietary intake. Why? Because the body treats alcohol like sugar and, at this stage, you are still boosting your metabolism for ultimate weight loss results and you need to keep blood sugars balanced.

If you do want to consume more alcohol (say, 4 glasses of wine per week), then on the days you do consume more, drop the grain option. Although grain and alcohol are nutritionally different, in order to ensure you hit your weight loss goals, they can be swapped on occasion.

Q: What is the healthiest type of alcohol to drink?

A: When considering alcohol, it is not necessarily the calories that are bad. As you can see from the table that follows, a glass of wine, a mixed drink and a beer are generally fairly close in calorie count.

The issue with alcohol is that it can make fat oxidation sluggish, leading to poor weight loss results. In fact, according to research published in the *American Journal of Clinical Nutrition,* fat metabolism dropped by a massive 73% for several hours following consumption of 2 drinks of vodka!

When it comes to choosing alcohol, the worst type, with a high fat content and lots of calories, is anything creamy—eggnog or Irish coffee, for example. There is no "best" alcohol to drink; however, red wine is rich in heart-healthy antioxidants. When consumed in moderation, it can benefit both men and women.

Calories in Alcohol

BEVERAGE	SERVING SIZE	CALORIES
Wine and champagne		
Red wine	6 oz (175 mL) glass	119
Red wine	8 oz (250 mL) glass	170
Red wine	26 oz (750 mL) bottle	510
White wine	6 oz (175 mL) glass	116
White wine	8 oz (250 mL) glass	165
White wine	26 oz (750 mL) bottle	495
Champagne	6 oz (175 mL) glass	133
Champagne	8 oz (250 mL) glass	190
Champagne	26 oz (750 mL) bottle	570
Mixed drinks		
Gin and tonic	Single shot*	120
Gin and tonic	Double shot	175
Vodka and cola	Single shot	120
Vodka and cola	Double shot	175
Bacardi and cola	Single shot	129

Bacardi and cola	Double shot	194
Jack Daniels and cola	Single shot	129
Jack Daniels and cola	Double shot	193
Martini, extra dry	Single shot	48
Martini extra dry	Double shot	95
Beer		
Bud Ice	1/2 pint (10 oz)	114
Bud Ice	330 mL bottle	132
Bud Ice	1 pint (20 oz)	227
Heineken	1/2 pint (10 oz)	114
Heineken	330 mL bottle	110
Heineken	1 pint (20 oz)	227
Labatt Ice	1/2 pint (10 oz)	114
Labatt Ice	330 mL bottle	132
Labatt Ice	1 pint (20 oz)	227

*A single shot is typically 1 1/2 ounces, a double shot 3 ounces.
Source: www.hornetjuice.com/calories-alcohol.html

USE 1 FREE TICKET PER WEEK

When trying to take off excess weight, the absolute worst approach is one that makes you feel deprived. If you are walking around feeling deprived or hungry, you are doing it wrong and you are at risk of a food binge. That's why I always tell my clients that they have 1 free ticket to cash in per week on whatever they like. This can be having an extra alcoholic drink, eating a grain option for dinner or opting to throw in some extra fruit, fat or starchy vegetables. How you cash in your ticket is completely up to you. Now, of course, I am not saying you can use your ticket for a large fries and double burger at a fast food restaurant—that would be way too much. But you *can* save it for an upcoming party or social function, for example, where there will be some food you would like to try or where you would enjoy an extra glass of wine. Here are some suggestions for cashing in your ticket:

- 1 5-ounce (150 mL) glass of wine
- 1 regular beer
- 1 mixed drink (but avoid those mixed with sugary juice or pop)
- 1 extra starchy vegetable, such as a sweet potato
- 1 extra grain option
- 1 extra fruit option
- 1 extra fat option (e.g., 10 extra nuts)
- 1 extra ounce (30 g) of cheese

Now that you know about the additions in the BOOST! phase, let's discuss what to do if you hit a roadblock or the dreaded weight loss plateau.

THE DREADED PLATEAU

Weight loss rarely happens in a straight line. If you have ever tried to lose weight, you know there is that 1-week (or, heaven forbid, 2-week) period when you simply do not lose a pound. I realize the frustration of putting in a perfect week and not losing a pound makes you want to say "%#$ it"—but I urge you, don't throw in the towel. As difficult as it may seem, try to keep your emotional response to the reading on the scale out of the situation. All plateaus break, and this situation will indeed change. Instead of giving up or food binging, try to focus on how good you feel and take charge by implementing the steps that follow to break that plateau for good.

I can tell you that after practicing weight loss for many years, I have identified a trend where over 90% of my clients hit a plateau.

For some reason, around week 7 to 9 of the weight loss process, the body and metabolism tend to settle and hit an adaptation mode where weight loss slows temporarily. Can this be fixed? Of course—but you need to know how.

First, determine if you really have hit a standstill in your weight loss efforts. I highly recommend weighing yourself and measuring your inches once per week (and no more!) to monitor your process—this is what the Metabolism Boosting Tracking Chart is for. If for 2 weeks in a row you have not lost a pound and inches have not dropped, then yes, you have indeed hit a weight loss standstill and need to shake things up in order to break the adaptation mode your body is experiencing. In truth, the closer you get to your goal weight and the more comfortable your body becomes at its set point, the trickier it can be. Thus, in order to break a plateau, you must confuse your body by breaking the pattern. In other words, it is time for a metabolic shake-up.

Steps to implement to break a plateau include the following:

- **Make sure you are eating enough calories.** Your dietary intake should never drop below 1,000 calories per day. Women should be eating approximately 1,200 to 1,500 calories per day, while men need to consume approximately 1,500 to 1,800 calories per day to lose weight continuously. If you eat less than 1,000 calories per day on a long-term basis, your body will think it is starving and will stockpile fat for preservation. As mentioned earlier, although a few popular diets recommend an extreme low daily caloric intake (fewer than 600 to 800 calories per day), weight loss on these types of diets is not long lasting.

- **Zigzag your calories.** "Zigzagging your calories" is another way of saying "caloric cycling." The process involves varying your daily caloric intake while maintaining your weekly intake. In other words, instead of eating 1,300 calories per day, one day consume 1,500 calories and the next day consume 1,100 calories. This can be as easy as cutting back on some protein, dropping your grain one day or dropping your snack. Why does this work? It simply keeps the body guessing and elicits the change mode it requires to break a plateau.

- **Take a sugar holiday**. While your caloric intake may be just perfect, you could be eating all the wrong types of calories—those that are keeping the weight on. If you have hit a plateau, I encourage you to review your food journal to ensure you are not overdoing it on sugary foods, including chocolate, refined flours or alcohol. If you are overdoing it on sugar, you will be bouncing around your blood sugars and triggering too much of your fat-storage hormone, insulin. I also encourage you to start reading food labels to check their sugar content. Manufacturers are very good at sneaking sugar into a product to improve taste.

- **Make sure you are eating enough fat.** The amount of fat you are consuming has not changed from the BALANCE phase to the BOOST! phase. If you are cutting back on your fat for fear of not losing weight, this is not a good idea. The good type of fat that you are consuming in the form of certain oils, nuts and seeds will help, not hinder, your weight loss process. Again, review your food journal to ensure your "good" fat levels are high enough.

- **For 1 week, drop the grain.** Although you are permitted 1 grain per day during the BOOST! phase, if you have been stuck at a certain weight for over 2 weeks and cannot get the needle on the scale to move, try dropping your grain altogether for 1 week to see if it makes a difference. If you do have a grain sensitivity (i.e., sensitivity to wheat or gluten), eating the wrong type of grain for your system can make digestion sluggish and trigger a stalling of your weight loss.

- **Eliminate common food allergens.** Weight loss can stall if you are eating food items you are sensitive or allergic to. The most common food allergen to remove from your diet after wheat and gluten is dairy. This includes milk, cheese, yogurt, cottage cheese and all other milk-based products (e.g., whey protein powder). The majority of people who have a sensitivity to cow's milk protein can tolerate goat's milk quite well. Thus, a small amount of goat's cheese (say, 1 ounce/30 grams in an omelet or over a salad) may still be consumed.

- **Do a different exercise every 3 weeks.** The key to breaking a plateau is to confuse your body out of its adaptation mode. If you have been doing the exact same exercise routine for some time and are no longer reaping the results by losing weight or building muscle, it is time to switch it up. You can change your routine even slightly and see the benefits. For example, increase your cardiovascular workout by 10 minutes, start increasing the incline on your treadmill, target different muscle groups with different types of weights or sign up for a yoga or Pilates class (or follow along with a home DVD). The key is change. So if there is a muscle group or a type of exercise you tend to avoid ("I don't want to do triceps exercises because they hurt too much"), that is precisely the one you should focus on to break your plateau.

- **Watch your stress.** Elevated cortisol levels can dampen blood sugar response and thereby facilitate fat storage. If you are under a considerable amount of stress, try to exercise, meditate and journal to lower your cortisol response. In addition, continue eating healthy, but also consider taking a break from the scale for a week or two to deal with your stress and not get discouraged. Focus on the improvement in how you are feeling and on your new heightened energy levels.

- **Sleep well.** Faulty sleep patterns can also make weight loss much more difficult. Try going to bed at the same time each night, avoiding television or the computer half an hour before bedtime, sleeping in a dark room and wearing comfortable, loose clothing. Taking liquid magnesium and/or valerian root at bedtime may also be helpful. Look for these products at health food stores.

- **Give it time.** If you're following the dietary plan outlined above and exercising as well, time itself will also break a plateau. However, I truly believe that weight loss is both a physical and emotional journey and that seeing results is the key to sticking to your path and keeping your motivation high.

Many people find the plateau an intensely frustrating time and need to take action to break the trend. I completely understand and encourage you to implement any and all of the steps outlined here to get to the final finish line of your goal weight.

If these steps don't break the plateau, there is no harm in returning to the BALANCE phase for 5 to 10 days. This will surely fuel your metabolism's fire and get your pounds melting away again. If, after resuming the BALANCE phase, you still do not break your plateau, it is advisable to visit your doctor to get assessed. Blood work can be helpful in determining if there is a hormonal imbalance that is making weight loss difficult for you.

The good news is that once you break the plateau, you will likely enter that sweet spot of weight loss where you are again on a downward slope for a long period. Depending on how much weight you have to lose, your body may hit an adaptation mode a couple of times during your journey. Hang on—it is part of the process and the steps just listed will likely correct it.

COMMON QUESTIONS IN THE BOOST! PHASE

Q. Can I start to eat after dinner again or do I have to stick to free foods after dinner if I am hungry?

A: If you want to keep losing weight effectively, I would advise not eating after dinner, with the exception of the free foods (soup broth, starch-free vegetables, herbal tea and water). If you find you are struggling and are extremely hungry after dinner, try eating a small amount of protein (1 turkey slice, 1 hard-boiled egg) or eating your 1 extra fruit (a green apple, say) after dinner. Try brushing your teeth or popping a piece of aspartame-free gum into your mouth to curb a craving. (See www.drjoey.com for gum recommendations.)

Q: Oh no! I had a full cheat/food binge—what should I do?

A: So, you fell off the health wagon. First, let me assure you that this is completely normal and it happens to everyone. At this point, you can take one of two approaches: (1) continue food binging and throw all the success and dietary strategies you have implemented out the window (this typically results in feelings of frustration or self-loathing and cravings rushing back); or (2) acknowledge the cheat, see if you can identify your triggers and simply get back on track blame- and guilt-free to continue your journey toward success.

I highly recommend you choose option 2! Changing food behaviours takes practice and involves repetition. If this process were just about the food, it would be much easier. As life will have it, there are stressors (big and small) that can lead to self-soothing or self-sabotaging behaviours with food or alcohol. If you are having trouble getting back on track, seek out a weight loss buddy (a friend, spouse, sister, nutritionist). Simply having someone to report to daily will help you grab hold of the rung to success once again.

Q: What do I do when I eat out at a restaurant?

A: When you eat out at a restaurant, it is all about making better choices. Of course, you can certainly dine out while following the Metabolism Boosting Diet—I am not an advocate of changing social plans or avoiding situations because of food, as that does not teach us anything. It is critical to start dealing with any and all circumstances to prove to yourself that you can indeed do this. When eating out, just be conscious of what you are ordering and what is already on the table (e.g., bread). I have had several clients show me the menu of a restaurant they planned to go to so that they could decide ahead of time what to order. Going in with a plan gave them a far better chance of sticking to their diet and still enjoying the meal. During the BOOST! phase, if dining out, simply drop all grain options (bread, rice, quinoa, potatoes) and have a meal consisting of protein and vegetables (stir-fried, steamed, in a soup or in a salad). Always opt for dressing and cheese on the side so that you can control the amount of fat you consume.

Q: What if I am at a friend's house for dinner? I don't want to insult my host by not eating what has been prepared.

A: I completely understand wanting to be a polite guest and eating what is served to you. When you are in that social situation, the best option you have is to practice portion control. In other words, eat like the French. Try a little of everything and watch the quantity of what you are eating. There is no reason you must clean your plate—simply trying a few forkfuls of everything will still be a compliment to your host. Learn to eyeball portion sizes, keeping in mind that:

- 3 oz (90 g) of protein is the size of the palm of your hand (without the fingers and thumb)

- 1 grain serving is the size of a hockey puck
- vegetables are considered free food
- 1 tbsp (15 mL) oil or dressing is 1 functional fat unit

If you are dining at the home of a close friend and feel comfortable doing so, tell him or her that you are trying to lose weight, have done great thus far and are determined to keep it up. Seeking health is a noble venture and those close to you will lend their support and understanding.

Q: Do I need to continue food journaling while in the BOOST! phase?

A: Yes, I recommend you continue food journaling throughout the BOOST! phase. Research is very clear that those who food journal tend to lose more weight in the long run. The greatest effect of your food journaling is keeping you conscious of what you are eating. In other words, it keeps your "eye on the ball" to ensure you are making good choices and eating with awareness. By food journaling on a continual basis (for a minimum of 30 days and ideally longer), you will create permanent food changes that will result in a long-lasting shift. The sample Metabolism Boosting Food Journal on page 271 asks you to detail how you are feeling on a daily basis (energetic, deprived, cranky, happy?). By making the connection between food and your emotions (e.g., "I had a fight with my boyfriend and felt upset so I grabbed a few cookies" or "I ate on track today and feel energetic, confident and in charge"), you will uncover and discover your triggers and what works for you, and so will be able to improve your relationship with food. Many of my clients find it very beneficial to record how they are feeling emotionally, physically and even spiritually.

Now that you have an understanding of the BOOST! phase, you will be able to follow this approach until you hit your goal weight. You also have the tools you need should you hit a plateau or fall off the health wagon. When you reach your goal weight, you will be ready for the next stage—the final part of this journey—MAINTENANCE. Which means results forever!

7-DAY BOOST! MEAL PLAN—PHASE 2

DAY 1

Upon rising: Warm water with juice of 1/2 fresh lemon

Breakfast: Mango and Strawberry Cream Smoothie (page 223) or smoothie of your choice

Morning snack: Tomato and cucumber salad with low-fat ranch dressing or 1 apple

Lunch: Veggie and Chicken Whole-Grain Wrap: 1 whole-grain tortilla + 4 oz (125 g) chicken + 2 tbsp (30 mL) hummus + mustard (optional) + chopped tomato, cucumber and spinach

Afternoon snack: 12 almonds with a 100-gram container of plain yogurt

Dinner: 1 cup (250 mL) Turkey Chili (page 237) with steamed broccoli

After dinner: Free foods if desired

DAY 2

Upon rising: Warm water with juice of 1/2 fresh lemon

Breakfast: Scrambled eggs (1 egg + 1/4 cup/60 mL egg whites) served with tomato slices and 1/4 sliced avocado

Morning snack: 10 grapes with 1 oz (30 g) low-fat cheese

Lunch: Lox and Cream Cheese on a Whole-Grain Pita: 1 whole-wheat pita + 1 tbsp (15 mL) light cream cheese + 4 oz (125 g) smoked salmon. Serve with cut veggies on the side.

Afternoon snack: 1/4 cup (60 mL) edamame, or sliced green apple with a 100-gram container of plain yogurt

Dinner: Chicken and Spinach Stir-Fry: stir-fry 3 to 5 oz (90 to 150 g) cooked chicken with sliced bell peppers and onions + handful of spinach + a dash of soy sauce. Add freshly grated ginger for extra zing.

After dinner: Free foods if desired

DAY 3

Upon rising: Warm water with juice of 1/2 fresh lemon

Breakfast: Antioxidant Berry Blast (page 176) or smoothie of your choice

Morning snack: baby carrots with 2 tbsp (30 mL) hummus

Lunch: Quinoa Bowl (page 231) or tuna sandwich

Afternoon snack: 1/2 cup (125 mL) non-fat cottage cheese seasoned with freshly ground black pepper

Dinner: Veggielicious Miso Soup (page 183) served with 3 to 5 oz (90 to 150 g) cooked chicken breast or 1 hard-boiled egg

After dinner: Free foods if desired

DAY 4

Upon rising: Warm water with juice of 1/2 fresh lemon

Breakfast: cottage cheese topped with 1/2 cup (125 mL) fresh berries and 4 walnuts

Morning snack: 1/2 banana with 1 tbsp (15 mL) peanut butter

Lunch: Toasted Tomato and Chicken Sandwich (page 233)

Afternoon snack: 1 cup (250 mL) Crispy Kale Chips (page 253)

Dinner: Faux Pasta: 1 cup (250 mL) shirataki or zucchini noodles (see page 169–70) tossed with tomato sauce

After dinner: Free foods if desired

DAY 5

Upon rising: Warm water with juice of 1/2 fresh lemon

Breakfast: 1/2 cup (125 mL) low-fat Greek-style yogurt with 1/2 cup (125 mL) ripe papaya and 1 heaping tbsp (20 mL) ground flaxseed or chia seeds

Morning snack: 3 clementines

Lunch: Turkey and Goat's Cheese Wrap: 1 whole-grain tortilla + 3 to 4 slices of nitrate-free turkey + 1 oz (30 g) soft goat's cheese + chopped tomato

Afternoon snack: 1 small non-fat latte and 1 apple

Dinner: Easy Egg, Olive, Tomato and Green Bean Salad (page 232)

After dinner: Free foods if desired

DAY 6

Rising: Warm water with juice of 1/2 fresh lemon

Breakfast: Chocolate Peanut Butter and Banana Dream Smoothie (page 176) *or* 2 servings Anytime Egg Bake (page 180)

Morning snack: 1/2 cup (125 mL) blueberries

Lunch: 2 whole-grain Ryvita crackers + 4 oz (125 g) nitrate-free chicken slices + 2 slices tomato + 2 slices avocado + sea salt and freshly ground black pepper to taste

Afternoon snack: Handful of Energy Trail Mix (page 257)

Dinner: 1 veggie or chicken burger with side salad

After dinner: Free foods if desired

DAY 7

Upon rising: Warm water with juice of 1/2 fresh lemon

Breakfast: Healthy French Toast (page 226) *or* 1 High-Fibre Blueberry Spelt Muffin (page 258) with 1/2 cup (125 mL) yogurt

Morning snack: veggie sticks

Lunch: Large mixed greens salad topped with Mighty Miso Dressing (page 184) and 3 to 5 oz (90 to 150 g) cooked salmon

Afternoon snack: 1 sliced apple topped with 1 tbsp (15 mL) almond butter

Dinner: Low-Carb Nacholess Salad (page 238)

After dinner: Free foods if desired

BOOST! PHASE RECIPES

Banana Berry Blast Smoothie

Frozen bananas are the perfect addition to a morning smoothie, as they are naturally sweet and lend a thick, creamy consistency when blended. Peel the bananas and keep them frozen in halves in your freezer for the sake of convenience. (*Serves 1*)

1/2 banana
1/2 cup (125 mL) blueberries
1 scoop vanilla whey protein isolate powder
1 tsp (5 mL) ground flaxseed
1 cup (250 mL) unsweetened almond milk
Handful of crushed ice

Blend all ingredients together until smooth. Pour into a glass and enjoy.

Per serving: 374 calories, 37.2 g total fat, 6 g carbohydrates, 28 g protein, 9 g fibre, 15 g sugars

Mango and Strawberry Cream Smoothie

Fresh mangos are best in this smoothie, but they are not always in season or easy to find. During winter months, consider purchasing frozen mango chunks, readily available at grocery stores. (*Serves 1*)

1/2 cup (125 mL) frozen mango chunks
1/2 cup (125 mL) fresh or frozen strawberries
1 scoop vanilla whey protein isolate powder
1 tbsp (15 mL) ground flaxseed
1 cup (250 mL) skim milk
Handful of crushed ice

Blend all ingredients together until smooth. Pour into a glass and enjoy.

Per serving: 341 calories, 6 g total fat, 47 g carbohydrates, 28 g protein, 8 g fibre, 23 g sugars

Two-Minute Mango-Strawberry Cottage Cheese Crunch

If you don't like cottage cheese, use plain yogurt instead. (*Serves 1*)

3/4 cup (175 mL) cottage cheese (2% MF)
1/3 cup (75 mL) mango chunks
1/3 cup (75 mL) strawberries, sliced
5 to 6 walnuts, chopped

Mix cottage cheese with mango and strawberries. Sprinkle walnuts on top.

Per serving: 300 calories, 10 g total fat, 22 g carbohydrates, 27 g protein, 3 g fibre, 23 g sugars

Metabolism Boosting Cranberry Oat Granola

Use this tasty granola on top of yogurt for a naturally sweet crunch. For a variation, use quinoa flakes instead of the oats, toasting for an extra 20 minutes. (*Makes 8 cups or 2 L*)

3 cups (750 mL) large-flake oats
1/2 cup (125 mL) raw almonds, chopped
1 cup (250 mL) water
1/4 tsp (1 mL) salt
4 tbsp (65 mL) raw coconut butter
1 cup (250 mL) honey
1/2 cup (125 mL) hazelnuts, chopped
1/3 cup (75 mL) pumpkin seeds
1 cup (250 mL) dried cranberries (preferably juice-sweetened)
1 tbsp (15 mL) cinnamon

Preheat oven to 200°F (100°C).

Toast oats and almonds on a cookie sheet at 200°F (100°C) for about 20 minutes.

Meanwhile, bring water to a boil in a small saucepan and add salt, coconut butter and honey. Stir until dissolved. In a large bowl, combine the toasted oats and almonds with the hazelnuts, pumpkin seeds, cranberries and cinnamon. Add the wet ingredients and stir until the mixture clumps.

Distribute mixture evenly on the cookie sheet and bake for about 1 hour, or until dry and crispy.

Let cool, then store in an airtight container.

Per 3/4 cup (175 mL) serving: 346 calories, 14 g total fat, 53 g carbohydrates, 6 g protein, 5 g fibre, 34 g sugars

Healthy French Toast

This is a favourite Sunday morning recipe in my household. It's rich in omega-3s and made with low-GI sprouted-grain bread—you really cannot go wrong! (*Serves 1*)

1 omega-3 egg
1/4 cup (60 mL) egg whites
1/2 tsp (2 mL) cinnamon
2 tsp (10 mL) butter
1/2 cup (125 mL) strawberries, sliced
2 slices sprouted-grain bread

Beat egg and egg whites with cinnamon in a shallow bowl.

Heat 1 tsp (5 mL) of the butter in a small pot. Add strawberries and lightly sauté for 5 minutes.

Melt the remaining 1 tsp (5 mL) butter in a pan over medium heat. Dip bread into egg mixture, then place in pan and cook until browned on the bottom. Flip to cook the other side. When the second side is browned, transfer to a plate and top with strawberries.

Per serving: 285 calories, 15 g total fat, 26 g carbohydrates, 13 g protein, 2 g fibre, 4 g sugars

High-Fibre Cottage Cheese Crunch

If you are like me, you often need a breakfast option that can be prepared in 2 minutes or less. If this is the case, this recipe is for you. (*Serves 1*)

1/2 cup (125 mL) cottage cheese (1% MF) or yogurt (any flavour)
1/2 banana, sliced
1/2 cup (125 mL) high-fibre cereal

Top cottage cheese with banana slices and cereal.

Per serving: 222 calories,* 2 g total fat, 41 g carbohydrates, 18 g protein, 11 g fibre, 19 g sugars

*Calories calculated using All-Bran Bran Buds.

Oatmeal Egg-White Pancake

Pancakes can be made in a way that offers a punch of protein and fibre. If you want to switch this recipe up from time to time, feel free to top with fruit of your choice (blueberries or sliced strawberries work well). You can also occasionally drizzle a small amount of agave syrup over top. (*Serves 1*)

1/2 cup (125 mL) instant quick oats or old-fashioned oatmeal
3/4 cup (175 mL) water
3 large egg whites
Brown sugar or cinnamon, for sprinkling

Cook oatmeal with water, as directed on package.

Add egg whites to cooked oatmeal and stir with a fork.

Heat omelet-size non-stick pan over medium-high heat. Pour in mixture and cook until top is golden brown with bubbles, then carefully flip pancake over. When bottom is browned, remove pancake from pan and sprinkle lightly with brown sugar or cinnamon.

Per serving: 240 calories, 2 g total fat, 17 g protein, 37 g carbohydrates, 6 g fibre, 2 g sugars

Classic Hummus

If you prefer to make your own hummus rather than buying it prepared, this recipe is simple and a definite crowd pleaser. Tahini (sesame seed paste) can be found in grocery stores and health food stores and adds a creamy texture to the hummus. (*Serves 10*)

1 can (19 oz/540 mL) chickpeas, drained and rinsed
1/4 cup (60 mL) olive oil
1 small clove garlic
Zest and juice of 1/2 lemon
Sea salt and freshly ground black pepper
2 heaping tbsp (40 mL) tahini

In a food processor, combine all of the ingredients except tahini. When well blended, add tahini and adjust salt and pepper to your liking. Pulse a few times to mix.

Per serving: 137 calories, 10 g total fat, 12 g carbohydrates, 3 g protein, 2 g fibre, 0 g sugars

Creamy Salmon Dill Wrap

Interested in avoiding wrinkles and having your skin look its very best? If so, omega-3s are a must-have in your diet. When buying salmon, whether it be canned, frozen or fresh, opt for wild-source, as it tends to be higher in omega-3s. (*Serves 2*)

1 can (7 1/2 oz/215 g) salmon
Juice of 1/2 lemon
1/4 cup (60 mL) chopped celery
2 tsp (10 mL) low-fat mayonnaise
2 tsp (10 mL) chopped fresh dill
Sea salt and freshly ground black pepper
2 oz (60 g) soft goat's cheese
2 small whole-grain tortillas
1/2 cup (125 mL) chopped Romaine lettuce
1/4 cup (60 mL) diced tomato

Drain salmon. In a medium-size mixing bowl, combine salmon, lemon juice, celery, mayonnaise and dill. Season with salt and pepper, using a fork to mix thoroughly.

Spread goat's cheese over tortillas. Top each with salmon mixture, then lettuce and tomato. Fold wraps and serve.

Per serving: 330 calories, 15 g total fat, 19 g carbohydrates, 27 g protein, 2 g fibre, 0 g sugars

Quinoa Bowl

Although this recipe is absolutely delicious, you may find this serving quite filling, as I do. Feel free to split it in half. The goal is to eat until sufficiently sated, not stuffed. (*Serves 1*)

1/4 cup (60 mL) uncooked quinoa, well rinsed
1/2 cup (125 mL) water
1 cup (250 mL) mixed veggies, chopped (e.g., carrots, celery, zucchini, broccoli, bok choy, chard)
1 tbsp (15 mL) sesame, sunflower or pumpkins seeds
1 tbsp (15 mL) sauerkraut
1 tbsp (15 mL) tamari
2 tsp (10 mL) sesame or flaxseed oil, or to taste
3 oz (90 g) cooked chicken

Rinse quinoa well. In a pot, bring quinoa and water to a boil. Reduce heat to low and cook, covered with a tight-fitting lid, for 12 to 15 minutes, until water is absorbed. Remove from heat and let stand for about 3 minutes, then fluff with a fork.

In the meantime, chop veggies and toss into a steamer. Put veggies that take longer to steam in first (e.g., carrots and zucchini), let steam for a couple of minutes, then add the rest of the veggies except greens—leafy greens such as kale, chard and bok choy do not need very long in the steamer. When the veggies are almost done, take off heat, add greens and cover for 1 minute.

Transfer cooked quinoa to a bowl. Add the vegetables in a layer and top with sesame seeds. Drizzle tamari over top. Add sauerkraut and drizzle with oil. Top with cooked chicken.

Per serving: 440 calories, 18 g total fat, 41 g carbohydrates, 29 g protein, 6 g fibre, 4 g sugars

Easy Egg, Olive, Tomato and Green Bean Salad

This salad is a low-carb alternative to the traditional Salad Niçoise, which often contains carbohydrate-rich red potatoes. This version is also rich in fats and proteins, which will leave you feeling satisfied. To boost your protein intake even more, simply add one to two more egg whites. (*Serves 1*)

2 hard-boiled eggs, quartered
2 cups (500 mL) arugula
1/2 cup (125 mL) green beans, steamed and cooled
1/2 cup (125 mL) fresh grape tomatoes, halved
4 kalamata olives, pitted and sliced
1 tsp (5 mL) capers (optional)
2 tsp (10 mL) balsamic vinegar
2 tsp (10 mL) olive oil

Place all ingredients in a large bowl and mix well.

Per serving: 312 g calories, 22 g total fat, 15 g carbohydrates, 14 g protein, 3 g fibre, 3.5 g sugars

Toasted Tomato and Chicken Sandwich

(*Serves 1*)

1 tbsp (15 mL) low-fat mayo
2 slices whole-grain toast
2 tomato slices
2 to 3 leaves spinach
3 oz (90 g) thinly sliced cooked chicken
Sea salt and freshly ground black pepper

Spread mayo on one side of each slice of toast. Top one slice with tomatoes, spinach and chicken. Season with sea salt and pepper. Top sandwich with the second slice of toast.

Per serving: 279 calories, 1 g total fat, 28 g carbohydrates, 31 g protein, 4 g fibre, 5 g sugars

Toasted Almond and Mandarin Quinoa Salad

Enjoy 1 serving (about the size of your fist) of this salad as a side for a carbohydrate option at lunch. Although quinoa contains a powerful protein punch, it is considered a carbohydrate in the BOOST! phase. (*Serves 8*)

2 cups (500 mL) uncooked quinoa, well rinsed
3 cups (750 mL) water
1 cup (250 mL) mandarin orange segments
1 red bell pepper, cut into thin strips
1 bunch green onions, chopped
1/4 cup (60 mL) slivered almonds, lightly toasted

Dressing
1/2 cup (125 mL) orange juice
1 large seedless orange, peel and pith discarded, and roughly chopped
1 tbsp (15 mL) finely chopped cilantro
1 tsp (5 mL) minced ginger
1 tsp (5 mL) sesame oil

In a pot, bring quinoa and water to a boil, cover with a tight-fitting lid and simmer for 12 to 15 minutes, until water is absorbed. Remove from heat and let stand for about 3 minutes, then fluff with a fork and transfer to a serving bowl. Stir in orange segments, bell pepper, green onions and toasted almonds.

In the meantime, in a small pot, combine all dressing ingredients and bring to a boil, then reduce heat and let simmer for 10 minutes. Drizzle warm dressing over quinoa mixture.

Per serving: 202 calories, 4 g total fat, 35 g carbohydrates, 7 g protein, 3 g fibre, 7 g sugars

Stir-Fried Tofu with Ginger Broccoli

A lot of the taste from this recipe is derived from the low-sodium tamari. Tamari is terrific for cooking, as it maintains its essential flavour even when exposed to high temperatures. In addition, tamari has approximately 37% more protein than soy sauce. As a lunch option, serve this dish with 1/2 cup (125 mL) quinoa or brown rice per serving. (*Serves 4*)

1 lb (500 g) extra-firm tofu
2 tbsp (30 mL) low-sodium tamari
2 tbsp (30 mL) olive oil
2 tsp (10 mL) fresh ginger, peeled and minced
3 cloves garlic, minced
2 green onions, diced
1 tbsp (15 mL) arrowroot or cornstarch
1/2 tsp (2 mL) cayenne pepper or hot sauce (optional)
2 cups (500 mL) broccoli florets
2 cups (500 mL) cremini mushrooms, sliced
1 red bell pepper, cut into thin strips
1/4 cup (60 mL) water
1 tsp (5 mL) sesame oil
Sea salt and freshly ground black pepper

Cut tofu into cubes and toss with tamari. Marinate for 5 to 10 minutes. In a large non-stick skillet, heat 1 tbsp (15 mL) of the olive oil over medium-high heat. Add ginger, garlic and green onions; stir-fry for 30 seconds. Drain tofu, reserving tamari, and add tofu to stir-fry for 2 minutes. Remove from pan and set aside.

In a small bowl, using a fork or small whisk, mix reserved tamari with arrowroot and cayenne. Set aside.

Heat remaining 1 tbsp (15 mL) olive oil in a wok over high heat.

Add broccoli, mushrooms and bell pepper; stir-fry for 2 minutes. Add water and bring to boil. Cover wok and reduce heat to medium, steaming vegetables about 5 minutes, until slightly tender. Return tofu to wok.

Stir tamari mixture with tofu and vegetables and cook until thickened and thoroughly heated; avoid overcooking vegetables. Add sesame oil and salt and pepper to taste.

Per serving: 283 calories, 15 g total fat, 25 g carbohydrates, 16 g protein, 3 g fibre, 3 g sugars

Turkey Chili

Of all the recipes we get feedback on in our clinic, this is definitely one of the top favourites. Filled with fibre and protein, this turkey chili is perfect on a cold winter day. Make your life a little easier and double-batch the recipe, then freeze in portion-size containers. This way, you will always have a home-cooked dinner waiting for you. (*Serves 4*)

1 lb (500 g) ground turkey
1 can (28 oz/796 mL) diced tomatoes
1 can (28 oz/796 mL) tomato sauce
1/2 medium onion, diced
2 celery sticks, diced
2 carrots, diced
1 cup (250 mL) sliced mushrooms
3 cloves garlic, minced
1/2 tsp (2 mL) each dried basil, parsley and oregano
1/2 tsp (2 mL) cinnamon
1 tbsp (15 mL) chili powder
1 bay leaf
1 can (19 oz/540 mL) kidney beans, drained and rinsed

In a large pot, cook turkey over medium heat until no longer pink. Drain off fat. Stir in tomatoes, tomato sauce, vegetables and spices. Simmer, uncovered, for 40 minutes, stirring occasionally. Add kidney beans and simmer for another 5 minutes. Remove bay leaf and serve.

Per serving: 371 calories, 11 g total fat, 36 g carbohydrates, 32 g protein, 11 g fibre, 12 g sugars

Low-Carb Nacholess Salad

In university, my go-to appetizer was a big plate of nachos. Not anymore! Unfortunately, most nacho platters are filled with saturated fats, calories and carbohydrates. So, in order to enjoy my favourite appetizer, I have come up with a low-carb nacho salad that truly delivers the same taste. (*Serves 2*)

1 1/2 cups (375 mL) shredded iceberg lettuce
1/2 lb (250 g) cooked ground chicken
1/2 cup (125 mL) sliced black olives
1/2 cup (125 mL) chopped tomatoes
1/4 cup (60 mL) chopped green onions
1/2 cup (125 mL) shredded low-fat mozzarella cheese

On a foil-lined baking pan, spread a layer of shredded lettuce. Distribute chicken, olives, tomatoes and green onions. Sprinkle with cheese, then broil in oven for 3 minutes or until cheese is bubbling. Remove immediately and transfer to a serving plate. Serve with guacamole or low-fat cottage cheese if desired. For a little crunch in your salad, break up 3 to 4 baked nacho chips over top.

Per serving: 448 calories, 31 g total fat, 7 g carbohydrates, 33 g protein, 1 g fibre, 2 g sugars

Watermelon Popsicles

Looking to curb your sweet tooth in a naturally delicious and low-calorie way? I recommend keeping frozen popsicles on hand as a sweet snack when wanting to nosh at night. Or enjoy when you are looking for a cooling, tasty and healthy treat. (*Serves* 6)

3 cups (750 mL) cubed frozen watermelon

Blend watermelon in a blender or food processor until smooth. Pour into a popsicle mould for 6, then freeze until solid.

Per popsicle: 24 calories, 0.5 g total fat, 5 g carbohydrates, 0.5 g protein, 0.5 g fibre, 5 g sugars

CHAPTER 9

PHASE 3: MAINTENANCE—RESULTS FOREVER

When diet is wrong, medicine is of no use.
When diet is correct, medicine is of no need.
—Ayurvedic proverb

At this stage of your weight loss journey, you have likely hit your goal weight or are within striking distance of it. For starters—bravo! I am confident you now feel much lighter, more energetic and have a surge of health that is priceless. This is also the time when many people ask the age-old question "I did it—but how do I keep it off?" There is almost a fear that you will lose control and gain back the weight. I assure you, there is no reason to worry. By implementing the steps outlined in this chapter, steps that involve both physical and emotional elements, you will be well equipped to keep the weight off for life no matter what events or stressors you encounter. One of my greatest joys is bumping into a former weight loss client two to three years after he or she has completed the program and seeing that that person still looks as healthy, svelte and fantastic as ever. When this happens I know they have lost their weight for good.

MEET THE NEW YOU

When you do lose weight to the point where you need to buy new clothes, it is likely that people have started to notice how great you look and are paying you compliments. While this is a wonderful thing, it is not uncommon to feel uncomfortable with it at first. You may feel pressure to keep the weight off, accompanied by your own concern of "Can I do it?" Your apprehension is likely especially high if in the past you were a chronic yo-yo dieter and have had an unhealthy relationship with food.

Consider the story of one of my dearest clients, Barb. Barb first came to me incredibly lethargic, wary about starting a program and feeling as though she was in a fog. To make a long story short, by following the Metabolism Boosting Diet, Barb lost a substantial amount of weight (68 pounds—see the photos that follow). After she had lost the weight and was looking fabulous, she opened up to me about being nervous about whether she could keep it off. Everyone (and I mean everyone!) noticed how fantastic Barb was looking—she literally was the talk of the neighbourhood. Understanding that Barb was nervous about gaining the weight back, I carefully went through the MAINTENANCE principles with her. Taking the weight off was one thing; keeping it off meant integrating a new set of principles into her lifestyle, which included family, travel and dining out.

I assured Barb that the MAINTENANCE tools would keep her on track and that, by sticking to certain principles, her success would be permanent and guaranteed. I told Barb that if she felt her weight creeping up slightly and her food behaviours changing (say, nighttime eating or eating sweets), to instantly refer to the MAINTENANCE principles to get back on track fast. I knew that going forward, the longer she was at her new weight, feeling healthy and energetic, the more comfortable she would be in her new skin.

Barb lost
68 pounds!

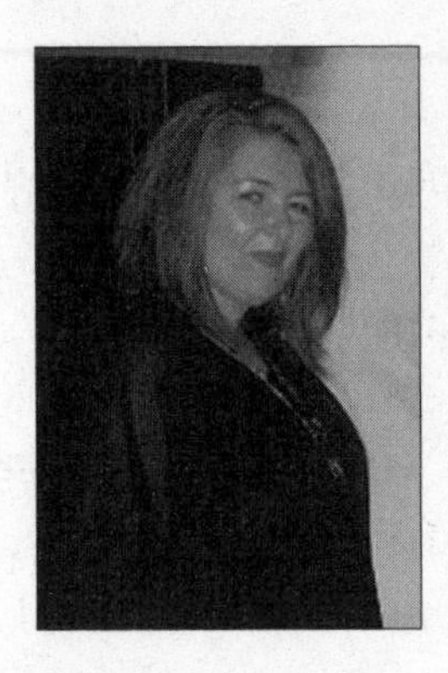

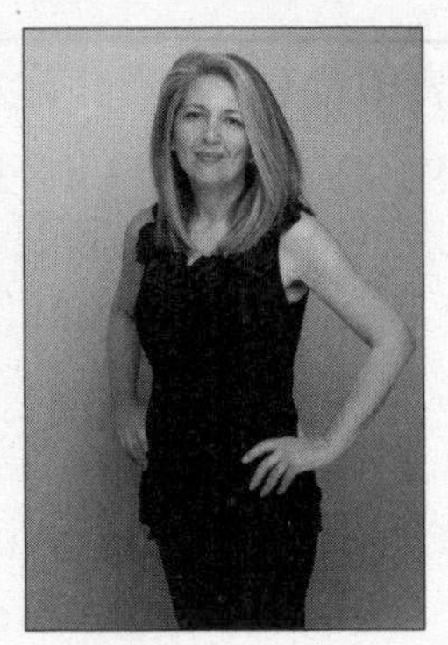

The entire goal of the weight loss journey you are about to complete is to create a permanent change for life. That is why the final step of MAINTENANCE is so important.

Before we get into the nitty-gritty of MAINTENANCE, let's first deal with any apprehensions you may have. Instead of feeling worried about *if* you can keep the weight off, feel comforted that the steps outlined in this chapter are going to be your lifelong go-to tools to implement at any time—when dining out, feeling stressed, working late or just sliding back into old eating patterns. Whenever possible, try to surround yourself with people who support your desire to remain thin and healthy, whether it be family members, friends, your nutritionist or members of your gym.

In addition, if you do feel outside pressures to eat more, drink more, party more, remember how great you feel at this moment. As you will see, a little bit of indulging is just fine, but overdoing it for a prolonged period can set you back. Hold on to this feeling of health so you never want to give it up.

MAINTENANCE PRINCIPLES

The MAINTENANCE principles to be followed now that you have reached your goal weight are ones that can be part of a routine you can follow for life. When you slip nutrition-wise (which you will—everyone does), the principles outlined in the list that follows will ensure that you get back on track and keep the weight off, while still enjoying delicious food options.

- Do not deny yourself—follow the 80/20 guideline of eating
- Avoid diet foods
- Eat up to 2 grains per day—occasionally toss your grain into dinner
- Continue to eat large amounts of vegetables
- Consume 2 to 3 fruits daily
- Watch your nighttime eating patterns
- Engage in physical activity regularly
- Continue to weigh yourself 1 to 2 times per week
- Do not consume alcohol daily
- Change your idea of snacking
- Practice 1 day of light eating per week
- Keep your fluid intake high
- Take supplements regularly

DO NOT DENY YOURSELF—FOLLOW THE 80/20 GUIDELINE OF EATING

If you are at a party and you cannot stop eyeing the chips, I have a suggestion: eat some chips! The long-term goal is *not* to keep you in a state of deprivation for life—that is not the balance I want you to strike. The goal is to make peace with food so you can enjoy your indulgences, such as trying a bit of dessert, eating a few nachos or having an extra glass of wine. The key is to eat on track 80% of the time and allow yourself to indulge 20% of the time, such as on weekends and special occasions like birthdays. When you do treat yourself, simply make a mental note that you will get back on track the next day. I assure you, falling off the health wagon and indulging at 1 meal per week will still keep you in a MAINTENANCE mode. That said, be aware that the size of your indulgence does matter. Determine what your favourite thing is as a treat—extra alcohol, pizza, dessert?—and drink or eat it very slowly, enjoying every sip or bite.

If you are going on vacation and plan to indulge a little more, be conscious and compensate with a bit more exercise, drink more water and balance when you get back home. If you return from vacation without gaining any weight, you did a great job.

You will notice I tend not to use the word *cheating* when referring to eating decadent foods. You now have the control. So if you wish to try a piece of cookie or a small piece of dessert, enjoy—no cheating, no food guilt. Simply do not make it a daily pattern. Try to eat like the French do. One of the greatest reasons the French are, on average, thinner and have lower risk of heart attack than their North American counterparts is because they are master samplers. Their portion sizes are generally much smaller than ours, meaning they eat—sample—smaller amounts of foods. The French do not suffer from portion distortion as we do in North America. To eat less and still enjoy the occasional indulgence, try taking mini bites of food, use your utensils to slow down your eating and make your meal last as long as you possibly can.

AVOID DIET FOODS

There is a huge surge in popularity of 100-calorie portion-controlled snack foods for weight loss. Unfortunately, a majority of these foods are filled with processed sugars, making them high on the glycemic index, which triggers the urge to eat more, leading to the oversecretion on insulin and excess fat storage in the abdominal region. In short, I am not a big fan of these types of foods.

Oftentimes, portion-controlled, high-GI foods actually thwart weight loss efforts, rather than assisting them. I have had many clients report binging on 100-calorie food items such as chocolate bars or pretzels during times of stress or when bored in the evening—before they even realize it, they have consumed six bags of 100-calorie treats.

I am also not an advocate of consuming artificial sweeteners such as aspartame in any significant quantity. I have seen far too many people who struggle with their weight overconsume products filled with artificial sweeteners. Take, for example, my client Taryn, who, when she arrived at my clinic, was drinking five diet sodas a day. This busy and extremely active mother of four came to see me because she had 15 pounds to lose. Taryn's cravings were out of control, she was not drinking water and her energy was extremely low. Although she was a relatively healthy eater and an avid exerciser, her mood, energy and weight did not reflect this. What I suggested to her was to simply taper off (with the intention of completely eliminating) the diet sodas, replacing them with water. I also recommended a few supplements that would assist with stress and blood sugar balance and then told her to come back within 4 weeks' time. When I saw this woman just a month later, she was no longer drinking diet drinks, she was crave-free and down the 15 pounds she wanted to lose. In this case, all she needed was a little fine tuning.

Not only have symptoms such as headaches, migraines, dizziness and numbness been associated with large consumption of aspartame but studies also show it increases hunger and cravings. When aspartame is consumed, the brain "thinks" it is getting something sweet and satisfying. When it does not (because the food is calorie-free), you are left wanting more and more food. Animal studies show that rats given sweeteners steadily increase their caloric intake, increasing their body weight and fat over time.

EAT UP TO 2 GRAINS PER DAY—OCCASIONALLY TOSS YOUR GRAIN INTO DINNER

Whole grains are filled with lots of goodness—fibre, vitamins, phytonutrients and more—but overdoing it can cause weight gain. As we get older, our bodies require less grain, fewer calories and more nutrient-dense options (e.g., foods high in minerals and antioxidants). As a general MAINTENANCE principle, 1 to 2 grain selections per day maximum is recommended. If you find yourself gaining weight, simply cut back on a grain option. In addition, limiting the amount of grain you consume *in the evening* is advisable for weight maintenance. When explaining this principle to my weight loss clients, I often say, "Picture your grain option as a baseball. Ideally, it is best to toss that baseball back and forth between breakfast and lunch. However, on occasion, you can toss the baseball to dinner." So, for example, if pizza is your thing or you would love some rice with a stir-fry on the weekend or once during the week, go for it. If you find the number on the scale beginning to climb, reduce your evening grain intake.

As well, some people lose and maintain weight much more effectively by cutting down their grain intake even more. Many of my wheat-sensitive clients react poorly (experiencing bloating, weight gain, constipation) to most grains and as a general rule eat grain minimally. If you are wheat sensitive, I recommend that you stick to wheat-free, gluten-free breads, brown rice or quinoa. And if you do find the pounds start to increase with 2 grain options per day, stick to just 1.

CONTINUE TO EAT LARGE AMOUNTS OF VEGETABLES

Make an effort to consume vegetables a minimum of 3 to 5 times per day. I routinely tell my clients, "If you want to feel alive, you must eat alive foods on a regular basis." Vegetables are brimming with nutrients and antioxidants and become even more critical to overall health and wellness as we age. Going forward, all vegetables (with the exclusion of starchy ones) are considered as free food and can be consumed in unlimited quantities. As far as starchy vegetables go, on MAINTENANCE, you can consume them up to 2 to 3 times per week. To recap, 1 serving of a starchy vegetable is equivalent to:

- 1/2 cup (125 mL) beets
- 1/2 cup (125 mL) corn
- 1 small (the size of an average baseball) yam or sweet potato
- 1/2 cup (125 mL) squash

White potatoes should be saved as an occasional treat. Instead of mashed white potatoes, try the Cauliflower Mash (page 185); it's the perfect side.

CONSUME 2 TO 3 FRUITS DAILY

Fruit is filled with goodness (vitamins, minerals, fibre, water, antioxidants), but it's possible to actually eat too much fruit, which can hinder weight loss success. Over the years, I've seen many people go overboard on fruit, halting their weight loss results because their blood sugars are just too high. Fruit is a wonderful part of your daily intake and can be included in smoothies, on top of yogurt or as a snack; however, it is best to keep to 2 to 3 options per day. To recap, 1 serving of fruit is equivalent to:

- 1 apple
- 1/2 banana
- 1/2 cup (125 mL) berries
- 1/2 cup (125 mL) cantaloupe or honeydew chunks
- 1/2 cup (125 mL) cherries
- 3 clementines

- 1 grapefruit
- 1/2 cup (125 mL) grapes, red or green
- 1/2 cup (125 mL) mango chunks, fresh or frozen
- 1 orange
- 1 peach
- 1 pear
- 1 plum
- 1 pomegranate

In addition to these, in the MAINTENANCE phase, your fruit option may now also include:

- 1/2 cup (125 mL) pineapple chunks
- 1/2 cup (125 mL) watermelon chunks

It is best to save dried fruit, fruit juices, dates and figs for occasional treats because of their high sugar levels.

WATCH YOUR NIGHTTIME EATING PATTERNS

One of the most important rules of maintenance is to keep an eye on your evening eating patterns. If you find your sweet tooth is creeping back and you are opening cupboards at night to see what you can snack on, this is a red flag. What might seem as "just a couple of cookies" after dinner will quickly turn into a faulty nighttime eating pattern that will cause your cravings to rush back and your weight to slowly creep up. Of all the principles of the MAINTENANCE phase, this is the most important one. Most often, eating after dinner is often not an indication of true hunger; rather, it is a sign that something is going on emotionally (stress, boredom, fatigue, wanting a reward, etc.). I tell my clients, "Don't get weight loss cocky!" You still need to keep your eye on the ball and follow the principle of not consuming grains after dinner. Think back to why you gained the weight in the first place. Don't let those food behaviours sneak back in. If you have the urge to eat at night, opt for these foods:

- low-starch vegetables
- soup broth (chicken or vegetable broth)
- unsweetened applesauce (1/2 cup/125 mL)
- herbal tea
- 1 cup (250 mL) air-popped popcorn
- 1 green apple, sliced

ENGAGE IN PHYSICAL ACTIVITY REGULARLY

"Oh no, I cheated big time last night!" If that is the case, your safety net—or insurance factor—to avoid weight gain is exercise. The truth is, once or twice per week is simply not enough. To keep your energy and mood high and your weight down, engage in physical exercise (the high-intensity workout outlined in Chapter 7) a minimum of 3 to 5 times per week. As we age, our metabolism slows, we start to lose muscle mass and our "bank of calcium" becomes smaller and smaller. To keep your bones strong and your weight down, and to continue to keep your metabolism running at high speed, exercise is a must.

CONTINUE TO WEIGH YOURSELF 1 TO 2 TIMES PER WEEK

When it comes to weight loss, there is a balance between taking charge of your diet and health and not becoming overly obsessed with it. To remain in tune with your body and your weight during the MAINTENANCE phase, it is important to continue to weigh yourself on an accurate scale 1 or 2 times per week—and no more. Don't weigh yourself daily. By doing so, you will see fluctuations that are caused by the time of month, bloating, a meal eaten the night before that was high in sodium and so on. Weighing yourself 1 or 2 times per week (pick a day of the week that is your weigh-in day) will help you to properly assess and monitor your weight without being overly preoccupied with the number. Remember, to be consistent, weigh yourself at approximately the same time of day, wearing the same type of clothing.

DO NOT CONSUME ALCOHOL DAILY

Although some studies do show that drinking daily and in moderation (1 drink for women; 2 drinks for men) has no ill effect on overall health, I am not an advocate of daily drinking as part of a weight maintenance plan. Higher alcohol intake is associated with higher amounts of abdominal obesity and can contribute to cravings, bloating and lethargy. As a general rule, a maximum number of drinks per week is 6 for women and 8 for men, although fewer is better.

CHANGE YOUR IDEA OF SNACKING

Snacking is one of the greatest pleasures in life and is a part of your healthy maintenance program. However, instead of snacking on processed foods that trigger cravings and weight gain, choose healthier and even tastier options that the entire family can enjoy. At my home, we are big foodies and keep healthy, low-calorie food on hand for that ever-important afternoon snack and as something to grab when running to a meeting or out the door in the morning. Whether it is healthy protein bars, apples and cheese, yogurt and nuts, or vegetables and hummus, there is always something on hand.

To make your life a little easier, when making the healthy snack option recipes, make a double batch. I am also an advocate of always travelling with food—in the car, in your purse, in your carry-on bag. By doing so, you will have more control over your food choices and won't have to worry about going hungry. Buy portable containers and a lunch freezer bag—they'll come in very useful. Weight loss aside, if you do eat the wrong thing for your afternoon snack, not only will your waistline eventually suffer but you will experience a plummet of energy that is not ideal midday. See the recipes at the end of this chapter for healthy snack suggestions. You'll find more snack suggestions in Chapters 7 and 8.

PRACTICE 1 DAY OF LIGHT EATING PER WEEK

For years, I have advocated the practice of 1 day of light eating per week. Why? This very effective technique will help to keep your weight down and will give your digestive system a break—and time to cleanse and digest unwanted food materials. I have also found this to be a very helpful technique for clearing up bloating, constipation and lethargy. Eating lightly does not mean you have to fast or eat next to nothing. On the contrary, what I am suggesting is that for 1 day per week, eliminate grain, red meat and dairy (except for plain yogurt) from your diet, sticking instead to hydrating foods and beverages, lean proteins, high-fibre foods and fruits and vegetables. For example, your day might look like this:

Upon rising: Warm water with juice of 1/2 fresh lemon
Breakfast: 1/2 cup (125 mL) plain yogurt with a handful of blueberries and 1 tbsp (15 mL) ground flaxseed
Morning snack: 1 green apple
Lunch: Large bowl of chicken soup with cut vegetables or Free Weight Loss Soup (see page 181)
Afternoon snack: Carrots and celery sticks with 2 tbsp (30 mL) hummus
Dinner: 3 oz (90 g) salmon with Free Weight Loss Soup (page 181)

You do not have to practice your day of light eating on the weekend—it can be any day of the week that fits your schedule. After your day of light eating, simply go back to your regular schedule. If you have had a food binge or major holiday feast, consider implementing light eating days for 2 to 3 consecutive days.

KEEP YOUR FLUID INTAKE HIGH

Proper hydration is essential to keeping your weight off and your energy high. If this new habit starts to slip, start making a conscious effort to once again boost your intake of flat water and herbal teas. Continue to drink water with freshly squeezed lemon juice—it will act as a natural daily astringent to your digestive system and it is great for your skin too.

TAKE SUPPLEMENTS REGULARLY

Supplements of vitamins, minerals, essential fatty acids and so on are the nutritional safety net that will benefit your overall health and help to curb cravings and keep your weight down. As a general rule, the basic supplements I recommend using on a daily basis are these ones:

- a high-quality multivitamin and multimineral complex
- a vitamin D capsule
- a fish oil supplement
- a probiotics capsule
- a green powder or chlorophyll
- an initial metabolic boosting supplement

Of course, there are specific supplements that are suitable for specific conditions and health needs. See Appendix 5 to learn which supplements may be right for you. Visit www.drjoey.com for my favourite product recommendations.

And now, all you have left to do is to move on to the last part of this journey: Part III, The Perfect Ending.

MAINTENANCE PHASE RECIPES

Crispy Kale Chips

Instead of eating potato chips, try this virtually "free" snack. These chips are low in calories and high in antioxidants, beta carotene and fibre—how can you go wrong? (*Serves 2*)

1 bunch organic kale
2 tbsp (30 mL) extra-virgin olive oil
1 tsp (5 mL) apple cider or balsamic vinegar
1/2 to 1 tsp (2 to 5 mL) kosher or sea salt

Preheat oven to 400°F (200°C).

Rinse kale and pat dry with paper towel. Cut off stems and tear leafs off the rib. Discard the centre rib pieces.

In a large bowl, whisk together oil, vinegar and salt. Add kale and gently toss.

Divide kale among 2 parchment paper–lined baking sheets. Bake for 15 to 17 minutes, until crispy.

Per serving: 105 calories, 14 g total fat, 14 g carbohydrates, 4 g protein, 2 g fibre, 0 g sugars

Baked Sweet Potato Chips

Feel free to double-batch this recipe, as these tasty chips tend to go fast. (*Serves 4*)

2 large sweet potatoes
spices of your choice (garlic and salt is a good combo)

Preheat oven to 400°F (200°C).

Spray 2 baking sheets with olive oil or cooking spray.

Thinly slice sweet potatoes in a food processor or by hand; they should be no more than 1/8 inch (3 mm) thick—the thinner the better. Arrange slices on baking sheets so they don't overlap. Spray with a bit of oil and sprinkle with spices. (My kids love these with sea salt and vinegar!)

Bake chips until they begin to lightly brown, about 15 minutes. Transfer to a rack to cool before serving.

Per serving: 155 calories, 5 g total fat, 27 g carbohydrates, 7 g protein, 4 g fibre, 2 g sugars

Edamame Hummus

Enjoy this hummus on whole-grain crackers or with strips of cucumbers. Tahini is a sesame paste, available in most grocery and health food stores. (*Makes 2 1/4 cups or 310 mL*)

2 cups (500 mL) frozen shelled edamame, thawed
1/2 cup (125 mL) water (or chicken or vegetable stock)
1/4 cup (60 mL) tahini
Zest and juice of 1 lemon (approx. 3 tbsp/50 mL juice)
1 clove garlic, smashed
3/4 tsp (4 mL) kosher salt
1/2 tsp (2 mL) ground cumin
1/4 tsp (1 mL) ground coriander
3 tbsp (50 mL) sesame oil
1 tbsp (15 mL) fresh flat-leaf parsley, chopped
Sesame seeds, for sprinkling (optional)

Boil edamame in salted water for 4 to 5 minutes, then drain. In a food processor, purée edamame, water, tahini, lemon zest and juice, garlic, salt, cumin and coriander until smooth. With the motor running, slowly drizzle in 2 tbsp (30 mL) of the sesame oil and process until absorbed. Transfer to a small bowl, stir in the parsley and drizzle with the remaining 1 tbsp (15 mL) sesame oil. Garnish with a sprinkling of sesame seeds if desired.

Per 2 tbsp (30 mL) serving: 61 calories, 5 g total fat, 3 g carbohydrates, 2 g protein, 1 g fibre, 0 g sugars

Easy-Peasy Banana Flax Muffins

Like the name implies, these muffins are a cinch to make. You'll find quinoa flour at health food stores. (*Makes 12 muffins*)

2 cups (500 mL) mashed organic bananas (about 5)
1/4 cup (60 mL) organic raw cane sugar
1 egg, lightly beaten
1/2 cup (125 mL) unsweetened applesauce
1 tsp (5 mL) baking powder
1 tsp (5 mL) baking soda
1 cup (250 mL) quinoa flour
1/2 cup (125 mL) ground flaxseed
1/2 cup (125 mL) chopped walnuts

Preheat oven to 350°F (180°C).

In a bowl, mash bananas. Stir in sugar and egg. Add applesauce. Stir in baking powder, baking soda, quinoa flour, and ground flaxseed until just combined. Gently stir in walnuts.

Spoon batter into a 12-cup muffin tin (greased with fat of your choice, such as coconut oil or butter, or sprayed with non-stick cooking spray), filling each to three-quarters full. Bake for 25 to 30 minutes, or until skewer inserted in centre of a muffin comes out clean.

Per serving: 120 calories, 2.5 g total fat, 24 g carbohydrates, 3 g protein, 4 g fibre, 3 g sugars

Energy Trail Mix

A handful of this trail mix a day for an afternoon snack is a perfect way to fill up and keep your blood sugars balanced. Or create your own healthy version: check out the bulk section at your local health food store—you'll find a world of nutritional goodness. (*Serves 10*)

1/2 cup (125 mL) almonds
1/2 cup (125 mL) walnut pieces
1/2 cup (125 mL) pumpkin seeds
1/2 cup (125 mL) sunflower seeds
1/2 cup (125 mL) dark chocolate chips (70% or higher cocoa content)

Mix all ingredients together and store in a glass jar.

Per serving: 182 calories, 14 g total fat, 12 g carbohydrates, 4 g protein, 3 g fibre, 4 g sugars

High-Fibre Blueberry Spelt Muffins

Spelt, an ancestor of wheat, is considered an ancient grain. It is great for those who have wheat-related allergies. However, this tasty grain still contains gluten and is therefore not suitable for those who are gluten intolerant. Spelt has a higher amount of protein than wheat and so requires more kneading. Also, spelt will not rise as wheat does. If you want your muffins to expand like regular ones, use half whole-wheat flour and half whole-grain spelt flour. (*Makes 12 muffins*)

2 tbsp (30 mL) softened butter or canola oil
1/2 cup (125 mL) organic raw cane sugar
1/2 cup (125 mL) unsweetened applesauce
2 omega-3 eggs
1/2 cup (125 mL) orange juice
2 tsp (10 mL) vanilla extract
2 cups (500 mL) whole-grain spelt flour
1/4 cup (60 mL) ground flaxseed
2 tsp (10 mL) baking powder
1/4 tsp (1 mL) salt
2 cups (500 mL) fresh blueberries

Preheat oven to 350°F (180°C).

In a large bowl, combine butter and sugar. Stir in applesauce, eggs, orange juice and vanilla.

In another large bowl, combine flour, ground flaxseed, baking powder and salt. Add to butter mixture and mix until just combined. Gently stir in blueberries.

Spoon batter into a 12-cup muffin tin, greased with fat of your choice or sprayed with non-stick cooking spray, and bake for about 30 minutes, or until skewer inserted in the centre of a muffin comes out clean.

Per muffin: 160 calories, 5 g total fat, 28 g carbohydrates, 4 g protein, 5 g fibre, 9 g sugars

Whole-Grain Lemon Poppyseed Muffins

Muffins are what I refer to as "the great disguiser" because so many healthy and natural foods choices can be snuck into any muffin recipe. One of the easiest ways to boost the nutritional punch of your muffins is to choose the flours wisely. You can start by simply switching from refined white flour to whole-wheat flour, which has far more fibre, vitamins and minerals. (*Makes 12 muffins*)

2 cups (500 mL) whole-wheat flour
1/4 cup (60 mL) organic raw cane sugar
3 tbsp (50 mL) poppy seeds
2 tsp (10 mL) baking powder
1 tsp (5 mL) baking soda
1/4 tsp (1 mL) salt
1 egg
1 cup (250 mL) fat-free vanilla yogurt
1/4 cup (60 mL) canola oil
1/3 cup (75 mL) lemon juice
1 tbsp (15 mL) lemon zest
1 tsp (5 mL) lemon extract

Preheat oven to 400°F (200°C).

In a large bowl, whisk together dry ingredients.

In a medium bowl, mix together egg, yogurt, oil, lemon juice, zest and extract. Add dry ingredients and mix until just combined.

Spoon into a lined 12-cup muffin pan, greased with fat of your choice or sprayed with non-stick cooking spray. Bake for 15 to 18 minutes, or until skewer inserted in centre of a muffin comes out clean.

Per muffin: 158 calories, 7 g total fat, 21 g carbohydrates, 4.5 g protein, 2 g fibre, 8 g sugars

PART III
THE PERFECT ENDING

CHAPTER 10

LOSE THE WEIGHT, LIVE YOUR LIFE

We are never given a dream without the
power for it to come true.
—Richard Bach

I've said it before: the weight loss world has gone a little crazy. Certain programs currently on the market are unrealistic, impossible to follow long term and even dangerous. My main complaint about some of them is what they do to the psyche of the weight loss seeker. Multiple failed attempts on dietary approaches that are impossible to maintain can leave you feeling emotionally beat up. I see too many people who are on the verge of giving up because they have failed the weight loss battle for the umpteenth time.

The Metabolism Boosting Diet's approach to weight loss is based on my years of research and the clinical success I have had with clients of every age group. The difference—what causes results to stick—is that there are no shticks or gimmicks that you have to follow. In fact, the Metabolism Boosting Diet addresses the totality of weight loss—emotionally and physically. By taking the time to understand, implement and change your relationship with food, and to understand the impact food has on your blood sugars, mood and overall health, you will create a food and mood reaction that will result in lifelong change. If you should fall back into your old eating patterns from time to time, you will have the tools to quickly get back on track without a struggle.

YOUR 5-POUND ZONE OF SAFETY

When clients "graduate" from my clinic, I typically review with them their "5-pound barometer of safety." By this I am referring to the fact that we all have 5 pounds we constantly play around with—5 pounds up . . . 5 pounds down. However, if the 5-pound zone of safety is broken, this is a red flag that needs to be paid attention to. In other words, this is your first indication that you need to shift your focus back to your eating patterns and your exercise and stress levels. This is why, going forward, I recommend weighing yourself 1 to 2 times per week maximum. Once you lose weight and start feeling healthy, fit and strong, you become incredibly in tune with your body. You will find that you are able to notice even a 2- or 3-pound weight gain and feel the symptoms of eating "off." If you go on a week-long food binge, you will actually experience a food hangover, which can include bloating, puffy eyes, irritability, constipation, inability to focus and poor immune system function. Thus, as a general rule, once you break the 5-pound zone of safety, you must put the brakes on and reel your diet and habits back in.

Take a look at a few more Metabolism Boosting Diet success stories.

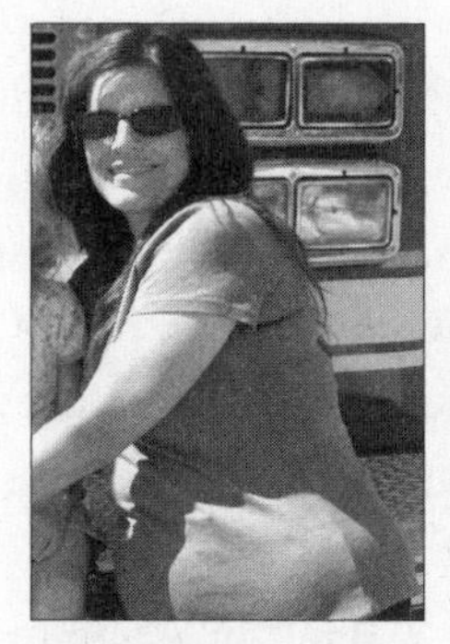

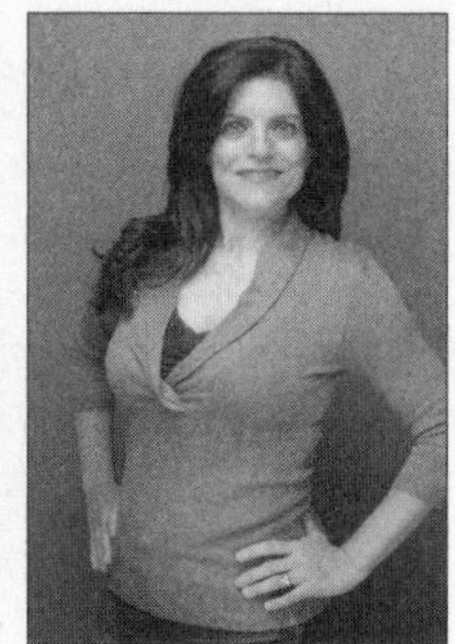

Mary lost
30 pounds!

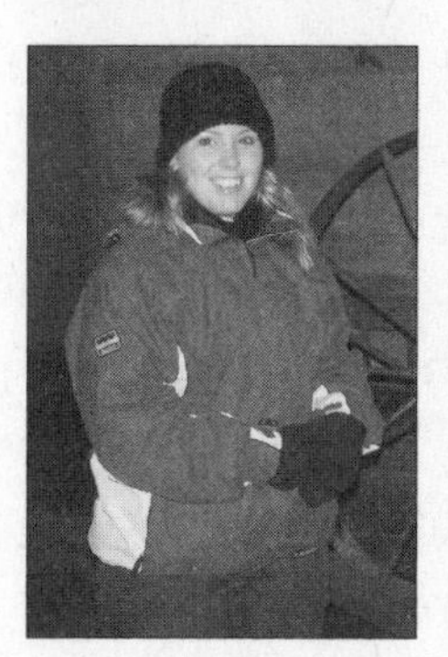

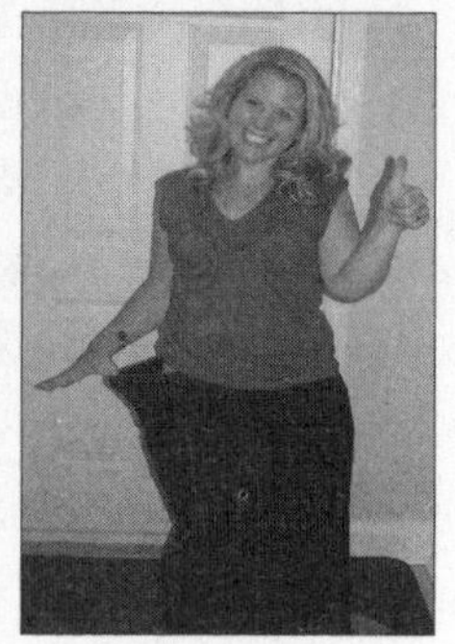

Tracey also
lost 30 pounds!

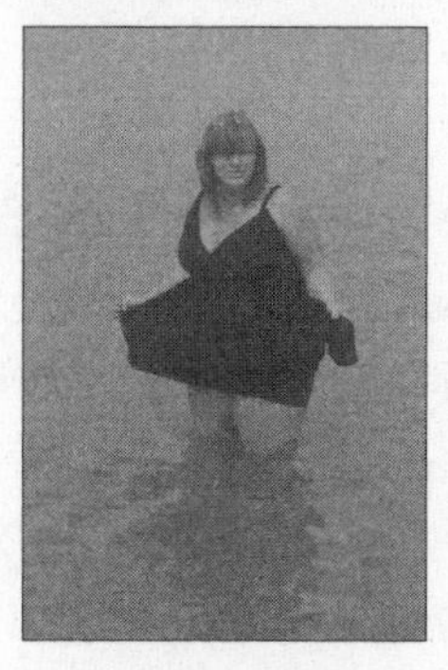

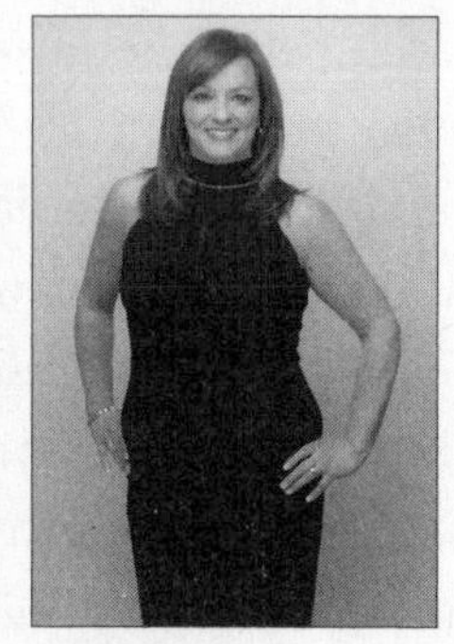

Josee—50
pounds down!

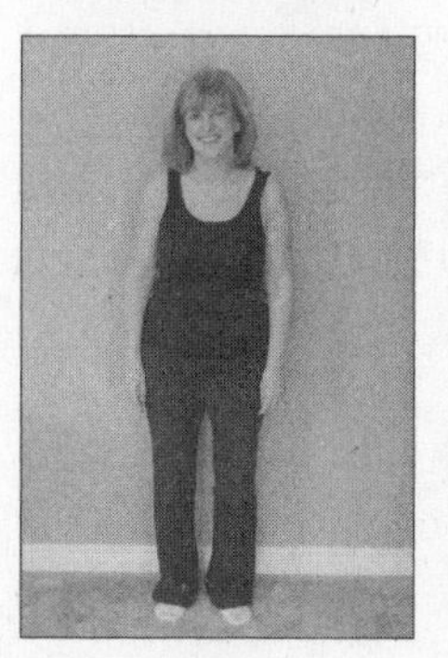

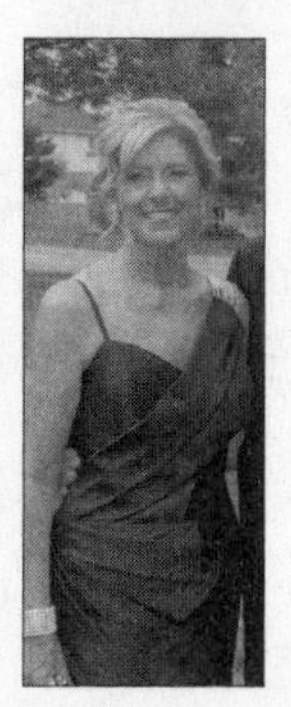

Valerie reduced
her weight by
25 pounds!

HOW DO I KNOW IF I HAVE NOW MADE PEACE WITH FOOD?

Most of us know what it's like to be injured and experience pain. The pain typically becomes a driving force and has a major influence on mood, energy and daily activities. The funny thing is, once you become pain-free, you quickly forget your previous state. If someone were to ask you how you feel, you might suddenly think, "Oh yeah, I don't hurt anymore!"

The same is true of weight loss. Back in Chapter 2, I describe how I get my weight loss clients to detail how they feel prior to beginning their weight loss journey (e.g., tired, stuffed, bloated). It is important to reflect back on how you felt before you began *your* journey to see how far you have come and how substantial your health changes have been. As I mentioned, I am also an advocate of keeping old pictures of yourself when you were heavier and hanging on to an old pair of pants that are now huge on you. This is a testament to just how significant your health changes are. Once you lose the weight and make peace with food, it is easy to forget just how lousy you felt before because you have slipped into your new self so beautifully.

It is common to feel a bit nervous once you have finally hit your goal weight. Allow me to offer you a little assurance by showing you that you have indeed successfully completed Phases 1 and 2 of the Metabolism Boosting Diet and have imprinted new successful behaviours for a lifetime of weight maintenance. You know you have shifted into a new zone of successful weight maintenance if:

- You feel hungry for breakfast.
- Food does not occupy all of your thoughts.
- You are in control no matter what life situation you enter.
- Your cravings are gone.

- Your energy does not fluctuate according to the food you are eating.
- Going out to a social function does not cause you to overeat, nor does it put you in panic mode.
- You are able to indulge and enjoy guilt-free (following the 80/20 guideline of eating).
- If you are not hungry, you are able to leave food on your plate.
- You still enjoy your food—and even more so!

So it's time to celebrate just how far you've come. And how far *have* you come? Simply answer the success questions that follow to find out. I applaud you on any and all health changes you have achieved, from lowering your cholesterol or no longer needing acid reflux medication to improving your mood and reducing your anxiety. It does not matter if you lost 5 pounds or 100 pounds—it all counts. And, whether you know it or not, you have inspired others to take the initiative to improve their overall health and wellness and to make the shift themselves.

Your success questions

My total weight loss is: ______________________________

My total inch loss is (waist, hips, chest):____________________________

When I began this journey my goals were to:_________________________

____

The way I feel now is: ____

The reason I want to keep the weight off is: ___________________________

At last, you have made peace with food.

Finally, before we end our journey together, I want to leave you with a few little reminders that will be helpful for future health choices and to ensure you are in the safety zone of weight maintenance.

KEEP YOUR EYE ON THE BALL

When my clients complete their weight loss program, I always say to them, "Now listen, do not get weight-loss cocky!" In other words, do not start thinking you can get away with eating refined flours or sugars, or with overindulging at night or with too much alcohol, without repercussions. Yes, you can indulge when the urge strikes, but . . . you cannot make faulty eating patterns a regular thing. The key is to eat on track 80% of the time and allow yourself to indulge 20% of the time. By following the 80/20 guideline, you will remain in MAINTENANCE mode and will easily stay within the 5-pound zone of safety.

WATCH OUT FOR THE DIET SABOTEURS

Over my years in practice, I have heard many tales of loved ones, friends and colleagues who have given my clients a hard time for making healthier food choices and wanting to lose weight. The ribbing typically falls under the vein of "Come on, you're no fun . . . live a little and eat!" While some diet saboteurs (cleverly disguised as your mom, your partner or your co-worker) are merely doing this in jest or wanting to share with you, it is essential to stay rooted in what is important to you. If *you* decide that it is a good time to indulge and treat yourself, then go ahead and enjoy. But try not to overeat simply because you are feeling pressure. This practice often leads down the path of unconscious eating and food guilt. Enjoy when you want to, indulge when you decide to and stay on track when it feels right to you—that is the key.

EVERY SO OFTEN, START FOOD JOURNALING AGAIN

To keep focused and to ensure you are still on track, every so often restart your food journal, detailing what you are eating on a daily basis. This practice is especially important for those of us who are emotional eaters. It is very easy to start eating because of stress or boredom. I tell my clients openly that years ago, when a loved one of mine was in the hospital for a week, I gained 10 pounds. Why? Simply because eating was the only self-soothing behaviour I knew to turn to. Food journaling will snap you back into awareness eating and will help you to make better choices. In addition to detailing your daily food, supplement and water intake, remember to answer the food journal question "How do you feel today?"

EAT SLOWLY

If you are a gobbler, you likely finish your meal in under 7 minutes, maybe even under 5. In addition to being overtaxing on the digestive system, eating too quickly tends to lead to overeating. When consuming a meal, it takes the brain a minimum of 20 minutes to register a full sensation in the stomach. To slow things down, take smaller bites, chew your food more (this takes practice and focus) and use your utensils slowly. As much as you possibly can, avoid eating at your desk or in front of the TV or computer screen.

FINISH YOUR DAY OFF AS WELL AS YOU START IT

Keep checking in with yourself on your daily eating patterns. Make sure that your eating patterns from 3 to 4 p.m. onward are just as clean as when you started your day. I have seen too many clients be on track with their meals at breakfast and lunch, only to let it all fall apart food-wise by the afternoon and beyond. Plan for your afternoon snack and enjoy it. The body has a natural blood sugar dip between 3 and 4 p.m., so it is important to eat a sensible afternoon snack to avoid entering the dinner hour feeling starving.

DON'T SAY _____ IT (FILL IN YOUR OWN EXPLETIVE!)

If you happen to fall off the health wagon, try not to crash the entire cart. In other words, don't think, "I just ruined everything, I might as well eat whatever I like." Simply enjoy your treats, watch portion size, and balance with a good workout or light eating the next day. If your cravings have rushed back in (which happens when you repeatedly overindulge), you need to take a sugar holiday and go clean again (i.e., return to the BALANCE stage).

TAKE CARE OF YOU

Be proud of all that you have done so far. Taking a health initiative and becoming your best self inside and out takes courage, strength and dedication. You have come this far; I encourage you to continue to make yourself a priority and keep yourself on your list. In other words . . . take care of you.

Remember, according to nutritional pioneer Adelle Davis, "We are indeed much more than what we eat, but what we eat can help us to become much more than who we are."

Wishing you future health and happiness,
Dr. Joey

METABOLISM BOOSTING FOOD JOURNAL

Date ____________________

Day # ____________________

Breakfast ____

Snack ____

Lunch ____

Snack ____

Dinner ____

How do you feel today? ____________________________

____

____

Water intake

Vitamins ____

For a free Metabolism Boosting Food Journal, visit www.drjoey.com and click on *The Metabolism Boosting Diet.*

METABOLISM BOOSTING TRACKING CHART

Starting weight ______________

Waist ______________

Hip ______________

Chest ______________

Week #	Weight	Waist	Hips	Chest	Total weight lost	Total inches lost

APPENDIX 1

YOUR NUTRITIONAL QUESTIONS ANSWERED

Many of us have "nutritionally burning" questions we have always wanted answers to. Keep in mind that nutrition is a vast field to which new research and information are constantly being added. We really have just begun to understand the enormous impact that food and eating behaviours can have on long-term health and wellness. Nevertheless, along my travels for work and in my clinical practice, I tend to hear the same nutritional questions. I'll address some of the most common ones here.

Q: Along with weight loss, I really want to improve the look of my skin. Is there anything natural that can help?

A: Yes, certainly. Your skin is the body's largest organ and is often a reflection of inner health. If you would like to improve the overall look of your skin (and appear 10 years younger!), follow the Metabolism Boosting Diet's 7-step skin protocol:

1. **Supplement with fish oils.** Fish oils condition your skin similar to the way hair conditioner works on hair follicles. When you supplement with fish oil on a regular basis, it improves the skin's moisture and texture. You will see reductions in fine lines and other signs of aging.

I highly recommend a distilled fish oil supplement (approximately 2 to 3 grams per day). When purchasing a fish oil, select a daily one that is enteric coated and made from smaller fish such as anchovies and sardines—the smaller the fish, the shorter their lifespan and the less accumulation of toxins. If the thought of fish oil brings back memories of your grandmother forcing you to take horrible-tasting cod-liver oil, take heart—fish oils have come a long way. You can purchase fish oils that are either in capsule form and tasteless or in liquid form and flavoured. Visit www.drjoey.com for recommendations.

2. **Eat vitamin E–rich foods.** Vitamin E is a fat-soluble vitamin that has been shown to prevent cell damage from free radicals and protect your skin against ultraviolet light. Sunflower seeds, almonds, mustard greens, turnip greens, chard and spinach are excellent sources of vitamin E. Vitamin E oil applied topically to the skin has also been shown to prevent skin damage from the sun. Sprinkle sunflower seeds over a salad or into a stir-fry for a delicious crunch and a vitamin E boost.

3. **Drink water with lemon.** In addition to helping you to lose weight and improve energy, drinking water with freshly squeezed lemon juice will hydrate the skin and reduce the signs of aging.

4. **Eat blueberries often.** According to US Department of Agriculture analyses, blueberries have 40% more antioxidant capacity than strawberries. Blueberries are high in vitamin C and can help strengthen collagen formation, reducing the signs of aging. Add blueberries to your morning breakfast or to a smoothie, or eat them on their own as a healthy snack.

5. **Eat vitamin C–rich foods.** Vitamin C is involved in collagen production and protects cells from free radical damage. Scientific studies show

that when lab animals eat vitamin C–fortified food, their skin is better able to fight off oxidative damage. Replenish your skin's vitamin C stores by eating plenty of vitamin C–rich fruits and vegetables on a daily basis. Good sources include bell peppers, oranges, strawberries, lemons and broccoli. I have also seen enormous benefits from applying a vitamin C serum topically. Anti-aging creams and serums that contain vitamin C (and also vitamin A) will keep your skin looking healthy and fresh as you get older. Visit www.drjoey.com for a fantastic skin-care line recommendation.

6. **Eat foods high in beta carotene.** Another antioxidant critical for skin health, beta carotene is converted to vitamin A in the body. Beta carotene/vitamin A is involved in the growth and repair of body tissues and may protect against sun damage. In extremely high doses, straight vitamin A from supplements can be toxic, so always avoid these. However, ample beta carotene can be found in orange foods like sweet potato, pumpkin, carrots, mangos and apricots.

7. **Gently exfoliate weekly.** Deep clean your skin twice a week with a gentle exfoliating scrub. This will remove the dead skin cells, allowing new cells to appear, giving you a more youthful look.

Q: I want to keep my energy as high as possible. Are there certain foods that promote an increase in overall energy?

A: Although there is no direct way to measure the effect on energy of specific foods, there is a scale known as the ORAC (Oxygen Radical Absorbance Capacity) scoring system, that measures the antioxidant capacity of a food. Foods high in antioxidants can help to release toxins and correct free radical damage (cellular damage), thereby improving overall energy and metabolic functioning.

A test-tube analysis first developed by the US Department of

Agriculture measures the total antioxidant power of foods and other chemical substances. The table that follows shows the top 20 ORAC-scoring foods.

Top 20 ORAC-Scoring Foods

Rank	Food	Serving size	Total antioxidant capacity per serving
1	Red beans (dried)	1/2 cup (125 mL)	13,727
2	Wild blueberries	1 cup (250 mL)	13,427
3	Red kidney beans (dried)	1/2 cup (125 mL)	13,259
4	Pinto beans	1/2 cup (125 mL)	11,864
5	Blueberries	1 cup (250 mL)	9,019
6	Cranberries (whole)	1 cup (250 mL)	8,983
7	Artichoke hearts (cooked)	1 cup (250 mL)	7,904
8	Blackberries	1 cup (250 mL)	7,701
9	Prunes (dried plums)	1/2 cup (125 mL)	7,291
10	Raspberries	1 cup (250 mL)	6,058
11	Strawberries	1 cup (250 mL)	5,938
12	Red Delicious apple	1	5,900
13	Granny Smith apple	1	5,381
14	Pecans	1 oz (30 g)	5,095
15	Sweet cherries	1 cup (250 mL)	4,873
16	Black plums	1	4,844
17	Russet potatoes (cooked)	1	4,649
18	Black beans (dried)	1/2 cup (125 mL)	4,181
19	Other plums	1	4,118
20	Gala apple	1	3,903

Source: http://www.ars.usda.gov/is/AR/archive/feb99/aging0299.htm.

In addition to the foods listed above, others that are energy boosters thanks to their water content, natural enzyme composition and ability to improve overall digestive capacity are:

- broccoli
- cherry tomatoes
- cucumber
- kale
- pineapple
- spinach
- watermelon

Q: There seems to be a lot of controversy over eating tuna and salmon. How can I enjoy these fish in a healthy manner?

A: There are pros and cons when it comes to eating fish these days. The pros are that fish are a wonderful source of protein and low in saturated fat. The cold-water type is a good source of omega-3 fatty acids. The cons of eating fish have to do with their toxicity level. With tuna, one of the most commonly eaten fish, the concern lies with the amount of mercury present. It is estimated that mercury levels in the environment have increased 3 to 5 times in the past century due to industrial operations such as pulp-and-paper processing, burning garbage and fossil fuels, mining operations and releases from dental offices. Mercury is an element that is toxic in all its forms. In fish, mercury appears in the form of methyl mercury, which can be very damaging to our nervous system when consumed. Effects can range from learning disorders and developmental delays to headaches, migraines, muscle aches, depression, memory loss, skin rashes and seizures. Mercury accumulation is of special concern for pregnant and nursing mothers because of the dangerous neurological effects mercury can have on fetuses and infants. Because of their longer lifespan, large predator fish, which feed on smaller fish, have a greater chance of accumulating methyl mercury than small fish.

In March 2004, the US Food and Drug Administration and the US Environmental Protection Agency announced their revised consumer advisory on fish and mercury consumption. Their recommendations were the following:

- Do not eat shark, swordfish, king mackerel or tilefish (large predator fish), as they contain high levels of mercury.
- Eat up to 12 ounces (375 g)—2 average meals—a week of a variety of fish and shellfish that are relatively low in mercury. Fish that are low in mercury are (canned) light tuna, salmon, pollock and catfish. Albacore (white) tuna has more mercury than canned light tuna. So, when choosing your 2 meals of fish and shellfish, you may eat up to 6 ounces (175 g)—1 average meal—of albacore tuna per week.

Salmon gets positive points for being a great source of protein and rich in omega-3 heart-healthy fats. However, according to several studies, farmed salmon contains unsafe levels of dioxins and PCBs, chemicals formed by unwanted by-products in a variety of industrial processes. PCBs are found throughout the environment and fish accumulate them mostly by eating other fish and fish feed. PCBs have not been used since the 1970s but are still lingering because they persist in the environment for several years. Dioxins and PCBs have been linked to several serious health conditions, such as liver damage, immune system suppression and developmental delay in children.

In order to enjoy the wonderful benefits of salmon, I recommend that you follow these guidelines:

- Buy wild salmon, which is available at most grocery stores. Wild salmon has fewer PCBs than farmed salmon.
- If eating farmed salmon, trim the fat off to reduce your exposure to PCBs. Also choose cooking methods such as baking, grilling or broiling over frying to eliminate PCB-containing fat.
- Choose canned salmon. Most canned salmon is made from wild fish.
- Eat farmed salmon a maximum of once per week.

Q: So what's the deal with soy?

A: Soy has been researched quite extensively, with a variety of conclusions. Thus, making your way through the soy controversy can be quite confusing, as the press has been mixed. As a general rule and as far as health and nutrition go, it is never a good idea to base recommendations on just one or two studies. I have come to realize that if you pick and choose research carefully enough, you can prove just about anything you like. The best approach, the one offering the least amount of bias, is to review the entire body of research and draw your own conclusion. Now, I realize you do not have the time to start poring over all the soy double-blind studies to make a decision, so allow me to summarize for you what the findings show.

Benefits of soy

- According to the US Food and Drug Administration, soy foods can help to lower "bad" cholesterol (LDL) and is good for heart health.
- Soy contains an impressive amount of isoflavones (phytochemicals found in plants), which have been shown to relieve certain menopausal symptoms, offer some cancer protection, slow and possibly reverse osteoporosis and reduce the risk of heart disease.
- Moderate soy consumption appears to reduce most types of cancers; its effect on estrogen-dominant breast cancers is unclear (see "Drawbacks of soy").

- People often choose soy as a healthier meal option—that is, instead of eating red meat—so in that regard it is beneficial.

Drawbacks of soy

- A very large percentage (over 90%) of soy is genetically modified and is heavily sprayed with herbicides and pesticides.
- Soybeans have an anti-nutrient called phytic acid, which can block the absorption of certain minerals, including magnesium, calcium, iron and zinc.
- The isoflavones in soy have a very weak phytoestrogenic effect (meaning they mimic estrogen). A growing body of research shows that eating a healthy diet that includes soy foods protects and lowers the risk of breast cancer, but the research is not clear for estrogen-positive breast cancers.
- Similar to dairy products, soy can cause allergenic reactions in some individuals.

Tips for eating soy in a healthy manner

- Always choose organic soy products.
- Choose fermented soy products. After a long fermentation process, the phytic acid levels in soy are reduced significantly. Here are a few examples of fermented soy products:

  Tempeh—a fermented soybean cake with a nutty flavour. Add to stir-fries or eat as a burger.

  Miso—a fermented soybean paste with a salty, buttery taste. Typically sold in plastic or glass containers, miso is readily available at health food stores. The type you purchase depends on your preference. Dark miso is much more flavourful than light miso and so is suitable for heavy dishes. Light miso has a more subtle flavour and works well in sauces, dips and soups. Miso can last in the fridge for up to 1 year (check expiry date).

Tamari (or shoyu)—a fermented soybean sauce, similar to soy sauce but thicker, that is very flavourful and salty.

For other soy options, I recommend trying to consume products that have undergone as little processing as possible (e.g., organic edamame). I am not an advocate of making highly processed soy "meats" and burgers or soy milk a regular part of the diet.

If you do have an estrogen-positive breast cancer, limit your soy intake to 2 or 3 selections of fermented soy products per week. The US National Cancer Institute and the American Cancer Society suggest that breast cancer survivors can safely consume moderate amounts of soy foods (a few servings per week).

Lastly, I am frequently asked, "Is soy safe for men to eat, given its weak estrogen-like effect?" Human studies have found that males who consume soy have had no changes in sperm count, quality or motility. Studies have also shown that soy isoflavones have no effect on circulating levels of testosterone or other reproductive hormones.

Q: I love muffins. Is it possible to eat them and still maintain my weight loss results?

A: Why, of course! Muffins are what I refer to as "the great disguiser" because so many healthy and natural foods choices can be snuck into any muffin recipe.

One of the easiest ways to boost the nutritional punch of your muffins is to choose the flours wisely. One simple switch is whole-grain flour instead of refined white flour; the whole-grain has far more fibre, vitamins and minerals. You can also try wheat-free flour options such as kamut or spelt, or gluten-free flours such as buckwheat, amaranth, brown rice or quinoa flour. I also recommend "punching up" the fibre in your muffins by adding 1 tbsp (15 mL) wheat germ or 1/4 cup (60 mL) ground flaxseed to the recipe.

To decrease the amount of fat in the muffins, use skim milk or non-fat yogurt. You can also substitute up to one-half of the fat in a recipe with unsweetened applesauce or heart-healthy olive oil.

As far as sugar goes, you can reduce the amount called for in most muffin recipes by half and not even notice the difference in taste. Or substitute with healthier sweeteners such as mashed bananas or add sweet spices such as cinnamon, vanilla, nutmeg or ginger.

Other wonderful muffin ingredients are nuts and seeds for their omega-3 value—try walnuts, almonds, pecans, sunflower seeds, ground flaxseed and chia seeds. Fruits such as berries, grated apples or pears, mashed bananas, dried cranberries and blueberries, and vegetables such as carrots or zucchini can also be added to boost vitamin and mineral intake. See the muffin recipes on pages 256, 258 and 259.

Q: What are the healthiest nuts to eat?

A: Several large-scale studies have shown that eating nuts can lower the risk of heart disease and is an important part of any weight loss program. Research has also shown that eating nuts is beneficial for lowering "bad" LDL cholesterol. In fact, in July 2003, the US Food and Drug Administration approved the following health claim for nut package labels: "Scientific evidence suggests, but does not prove, that eating 1.5 ounces per day of some nuts, as part of a diet low in saturated fat and cholesterol, may reduce the risk of heart disease."

Because nuts are so nutrient dense, it takes only a small handful to provide you with sustainable fuel and satisfy hunger (and help you stay feeling full longer), so you need to be conscious of portion control. The motto with nuts is "A little goes a long way."

Recommended portion sizes are as follows:

- 10 to 15 almonds
- 6 to 8 Brazil nuts
- 10 to 15 cashews
- 8 to 10 hazelnuts
- 10 macadamia nuts
- 15 to 20 peanuts
- 12 to 15 pecan halves
- 25 to 30 pistachios
- 7 to 10 walnut halves

If you do have trouble with portion control, simply dole out the allotted amount of nuts and put them in a container or resealable bag—handy for keeping in your purse or briefcase.

The healthiest nuts are these:

Walnuts. Of all nuts, walnuts offer the richest source of omega-3 fatty acids, which offer protection for your heart, help boost immunity, are anti-inflammatory, have shown beneficial effects on depression and can even assist with weight loss. In fact, studies at Loma Linda University in California showed that eating a few walnuts before a meal decreased appetite and caused people to eat less. Walnuts are also rich in protein, B vitamins, vitamin E, magnesium, calcium, potassium and manganese.

1 ounce (30 g) (about 14 halves): 185 calories, 18 grams of fat

Almonds. Just 1/4 cup (60 mL) of almonds contains your daily recommended amount of magnesium and contains 7 grams of protein and 4 grams of fibre. Almonds are also rich in vitamin E, potassium, manganese and calcium. In fact, 1/4 cup (60 mL) of almonds has almost as much calcium as the same amount of milk. Almonds have also been shown to be good for the colon and digestive health. With almost 70% of its fat being of the heart-healthy monounsaturated kind, almonds are very beneficial for keeping arteries in tiptop shape and lowering cholesterol levels.

1 ounce (30 g) (about 22 nuts): 170 calories, 15 grams of fat

Cashews. Cashews are rich in monounsaturated heart-healthy fat and are also a rich source of fibre (which fills you up). In addition, cashews are high in antioxidants, copper, magnesium, zinc, iron and biotin.

1 ounce (30 g) (16 to 18 nuts): 162 calories, 12 grams of fat

Pistachios. Pistachios, a snacking favourite, are a rich source of fibre, antioxidants, potassium, magnesium and vitamin B6. Containing mostly heart-healthy monounsaturated fat, pistachios are also rich in phytosterols, known for their cholesterol-lowering effects. According to a study published in the *Journal of the American College of Nutrition*, volunteers who followed a weight-reduction diet for 12 weeks and ate 2 ounces (60 g) of pistachios daily as an afternoon snack, instead of an equal amount of refined carbohydrates in the form of pretzels, lost weight and had lowered blood levels of heart-unhealthy triglycerides.

1 ounce (30 g) (about 45 nuts): 160 calories, 13 grams of fat

Pecans. Pecans are rich in numerous minerals and vitamins, including calcium, magnesium, copper, vitamins E and A, folic acid and several B vitamins. Pecans are a part of a heart-healthy diet, as they help to lower cholesterol levels. Pecans are also sodium-free, high in monounsaturated fat and a good source of protein and fibre. Simply add pieces to your salads and soups or serve with cooked meats for a rich taste.

1 ounce (30 g) (about 20 halves): 200 calories, 21 grams of fat

Macadamia nuts. Macadamia nuts provide a wide range of nutritional benefits. These crunchy nuts are a high-energy food and a rich source of protein, fibre and antioxidants. They are higher in monounsaturated fats than any other nut. Studies have shown that adding a modest amount of macadamia nuts to the diet significantly reduce cholesterol levels.

1 ounce (30 g) (10 to 12 nuts): 200 calories, 22 grams of fat

Brazil nuts. Brazil nuts are rich in fibre, protein, magnesium, vitamin E and selenium. Selenium is a powerful antioxidant that helps to neutralize cellular damage (a.k.a. free radical damage). Studies have shown the selenium found in Brazil nuts to be beneficial for preventing certain types of cancer, including breast cancer.

1 ounce (30 g) (6 to 8 nuts): 186 calories; 19 grams of fat

Peanuts. Peanuts are not actually nuts; rather, they're a member of the legume family and so related to lentils and beans. However, in the culinary world, they're classified as nuts. Peanuts contain a high amount of protein, are rich in monounsaturated fat and are a good source of coenzyme Q10, a powerful antioxidant proven to be essential in heart health and heart disease prevention. Peanuts also contain high levels of niacin (vitamin B3), which helps in the recovery of cellular damage and provides protection against Alzheimer's disease and age-related cognitive problems. Lastly, peanuts have a high resveratrol content. This bioflavonoid is believed to improve blood flow in the brain by as much as 30%, thus greatly reducing the risk of stroke. Studies showed that adding even small amounts of peanut products to the diet can reduce LDL (bad) cholesterol by 14%.

1 ounce (30 g) (about 22 nuts): 165 calories, 14 grams of fat

Q: I am having a lot of trouble regulating my sleep pattern, and I think it's affecting my weight loss progress. What can I do to get a decent night's sleep?

A: When I had my second child, lo and behold—she was colicky. For the first 3 months, the sleep deprivation I experienced was quite extreme, as I was awake every one and a half hours throughout the night. At the same time, I was eager to start losing my baby weight, as I had TV appearances coming up. Although in the past my metabolism typically responded to my weight loss regime by losing 2 to 4 pounds per week, this time was different. For the first 3 months, I was lucky if I lost a pound a week. Why was this time different? The stress and the extreme sleep deprivation I was experiencing were keeping the needle on the scale from moving. As soon as my little one settled in and my sleep patterns started to regulate, my pounds soon started melting away once again.

Poor sleep can interfere with the body's ability to metabolize carbohydrates. It can raise insulin levels and promote fat storage, drive down leptin levels, create cravings and increase hunger. It can increase blood pressure and the risk for heart disease.

The intimate relationship between proper sleep and weight loss has been documented in a variety of sleep and weight loss studies. In fact, one study showed that women who sleep 5 hours or less per night generally weigh more than women who sleep 7 hours per night. In addition to helping weight loss, sleeping well and establishing a regular sleep routine is critical for immune system functioning, mental health and proper repair of the body. When you sleep, your body actually works on restoring itself from the day's events, emotionally and physically. Over the years, I have seen dozens of shift workers struggle with mood and weight loss due to their ever-changing and disruptive sleep cycle.

You will find that once you have hit your target weight on the

Metabolism Boosting Diet, your sleep patterns improve dramatically. In fact, this is often one of the first improvements I hear about. However, if your healthful sleep pattern has been thrown off for a long time (thanks to hormonal imbalances, stress, travel or some other event), it may be a little difficult to get back on track. Be patient and consistent. By implementing the following steps, you will soon be on your way to a better night's sleep.

- Minimize your alcohol intake, as it can interfere with REM sleep.
- Do not eat a large evening meal, as it can disrupt sleep patterns.
- Do not drink a caffeinated beverage from 2 p.m. onward.
- Put 3 to 4 drops of essential lavender oil on your pillow before bedtime to induce a sense of calm and sleepiness.
- Try to clear up any conflict you may have before going to sleep—as my father always said, "Never go to sleep angry." If you cannot clear up the conflict, write your thoughts and feelings in your journal, or meditate to try to destress and relax.
- Create a calming sleep environment. Make sure your bedroom is completely dark and well ventilated. The ideal temperature for sleeping is between 65 and 70 degrees Fahrenheit (18 and 21 degrees Celsius). If in the wintertime you are affected by dry air, which makes sleep difficult, invest in a high-quality steam humidifier.
- Aim for a regular bedtime routine. In other words, try to fall asleep and wake at the same time each day (yes, even on the weekends).
- Avoid sleeping in too long, as it will create a groggy start to the day and will make falling sleeping in the evening even more difficult.
- Exercise regularly to reduce stress and body weight.
- If you do not fall asleep within half an hour of going to bed, get out of bed to read a book or write in your journal. Lying in bed not being able to fall asleep can create feelings of anxiety. It is best to break the cycle by engaging in another activity until you feel drowsy.

- If you are feeling tense or stressed, try practicing breathing exercises. With each breath you inhale, imagine you are breathing in happiness and positive energy; with each outgoing breath, imagine you are exhaling stress, worries and tension.
- As a general rule, try to go to bed by 10 p.m. According to Ayurvedic medicine, for a quality, deep sleep, it is critical not go to sleep too late in the evening. Also avoid stimulating TV or computer work before bedtime.
- Supplement with a minimum of 1,000 international units of vitamin D. Vitamin D has been shown to help improve sleep quality. In addition, allow your skin to be exposed to natural sunlight and eat foods high in vitamin D, such as oily fish like salmon, cod and mackerel; shrimp; and eggs and fortified milk.
- Supplement with calcium and magnesium. The sedative effect of calcium makes it one of the most effective vitamins for improving sleep quality. The recommended dose is 1,500 to 2,000 milligrams 1 hour before bedtime. Magnesium also has a calming effect on the brain and can help to bring on a good night's sleep. Liquid calcium and/or magnesium are ideal for increased absorption.
- Take a high-quality multi–B vitamin supplement. It can help to calm nerves.
- Supplement with time-released melatonin capsules. It is critical for the melatonin to be time-released for it to have the proper effect. Visit www.drjoey.com for product recommendations.

Q: *What about chocolate?*

A: Chocolate is one of the great pleasures of life and can indeed be incorporated into the Metabolism Boosting Diet. However, if you begin the program with a serious sweet tooth and identify yourself as a chronic chocoholic, it's best to eliminate chocolate during your BALANCE phase.

Once your sweet tooth has subsided, feel free to introduce dark chocolate back into your diet on a regular basis (1 to 2 squares per day). Dark chocolate (65% to 70% cocoa) is a greater source of flavonoids (antioxidants) than milk chocolate or white chocolate. Research has also shown that dark chocolate offers cardiovascular benefits and helps lower cholesterol by as much as 10%. However, chocolate is high in calories, so don't overdo it.

Q: How do I know if I am allergic, as opposed to sensitive, to a certain food?

A: Food allergies and food sensitivities cause very different reactions in the body that range in severity. A food *allergy* is typically an immediate response by the immune system in reaction to an offending food, usually protein. The body "thinks" the food in question is an invader or a threat; treating it as a poison, it launches an immune system attack. Symptoms can include swelling, itching, tingling, burning, rashes, hives, vomiting and diarrhea. True allergies can be detected by a skin scratch test or by RAST tests that measure the IgE antibodies in the blood. Unfortunately, these types of allergies are typically fixed for life. Food allergies often run in families and affect between 2% and 4% of adults and between 6% and 8% of children.

In Canada, there are nine priority food allergens (substances that cause allergies):

- peanuts
- tree nuts (almonds, Brazil nuts, cashews, hazelnuts, macadamia nuts, pecans, pine nuts, pistachios and walnuts)
- sesame seeds
- milk
- eggs

- fish (including shellfish and crustaceans)
- soy (including miso)
- wheat
- sulphites

A food *sensitivity* (intolerance), on the other hand, is typically a digestive system response rather than an immune system response. It occurs when something in a food—say, a protein in cow's milk—irritates the digestive system and the food is unable to be broken down. Unlike a food allergy, which causes an immediate reaction, food sensitivities can cause reactions in the body that show themselves within as little as 2 hours or as long as 2 days after ingesting the food. A wide variety of symptoms may be experienced, including fatigue, mood swings, depression, hyperactivity, gas, bloating, constipation, eczema, asthma, headache and sinus congestion. Food sensitivities can also cause cravings and sluggish weight loss results.

If you suspect you have a sensitivity or intolerance to a specific food, perhaps wheat or dairy, eliminate the food from your diet for a minimum of 2 weeks while noting your symptoms and whether they improve. Often, food sensitivities are not fixed and once diet is improved and the immune system is boosted and strengthened, you may be able to be reintroduce the offending food into your diet.

If you have other questions, simply e-mail me at www.drjoey.com—I would love to hear from you!

APPENDIX 2
LABEL READING

The Nutrition Facts table lists the amount of important nutrients and calories in a certain amount of food. This information, along with the % Daily Value, helps you to compare and choose foods. Almost all pre-packaged foods in Canada and the United States are required to carry a Nutrition Facts table.

Nutrition Facts Serving Size 1 cup (228 g) Servings Per Container 2	
Amount Per Serving	**% Daily Value**
Calories 250	
Fat 12 g	**18%**
Saturated Fat 3 g	**15%**
Trans Fat 3 g	
Cholesterol 30 mg	**10%**
Sodium 660 mg	**28%**
Total Carbohydrate 31 g	**10%**
Dietary Fiber 0 g	**0%**
Sugars 5 g	
Protein 5 g	
Vitamin A	**4%**
Vitamin C	**2%**
Calcium	**20%**
Iron	**2%**

SERVING SIZE. The product's serving size is located at the top of the table. These amounts are standardized for easier comparison with other food items. Serving sizes are provided in familiar units, such as cups or grams. Paying attention to serving size is of the utmost importance. Although a food item may appear lower in fat or calories, the serving size of the item might be quite small. In other words, you may typically eat up to 2 or even 3 times the serving size listed on the package, meaning you eat 2 or 3 times the amount of fat or number of calories listed.

CALORIES (KCAL). A calorie is a unit of energy and differs from food to food because of the different nutrient content. Calories listed on the Nutrition Facts table provide a measurement of how much energy you obtain after eating a serving size of a specific food. Review the calories closely. As we know now, labels such as "fat-free" or "sugar-free" do not necessarily mean the food in question is low in calories.

NUTRIENTS LISTED. This section of the Nutrition Facts table lists the weight of total fat, saturated and trans fats, cholesterol, carbohydrates (including fibre and added sugars) and protein in 1 serving of the food. Percent daily values (see list that follows) of these nutrients are also provided. Vitamins A and C, calcium and iron are expressed in percent daily values only. Other nutrients may be included if the manufacturer decides to do so. As of January 2006, all Nutrition Facts tables indicate the presence of trans fatty acids.

- **Total fat:** The weight of fat (in grams) in 1 serving of food.
- **Saturated fat:** The weight of saturated fat (in grams) in 1 serving of food.
- **Trans fat:** The weight of trans fat (in grams) in 1 serving of food.
- **Cholesterol:** The weight of cholesterol (in milligrams) in 1 serving of food.

- **Sodium:** The weight of sodium (in milligrams) in 1 serving of food.
- **Total carbohydrates:** The weight of both complex and simple carbohydrates (in grams) in 1 serving of food.
- **Dietary Fibre:** The weight of fibre (in grams) in 1 serving of food.
- **Sugars:** The weight of simple carbohydrates (in grams) in 1 serving of this food; to find out how many complex carbohydrates are in the food, simply subtract sugars from total carbohydrate.
- **Protein:** The weight of protein (in grams) in 1 serving of food.

PERCENT DAILY VALUES. These values provide an estimate of the percentage of a nutrient from 1 serving in a typical 2,000-calorie diet. Keep in mind the following:

- 5% or less of your daily recommended amount of a nutrient is considered a poor source of that nutrient.
- 10% to 20% is considered a good source of that nutrient.
- More than 20% is considered a high amount of that nutrient.

INGREDIENT LIST. In addition to the Nutrition Facts table, the ingredient list contains a lot of information. Ingredients are listed by weight from highest to lowest. Beware of foods whose first one or two ingredients are sugar (watch out for the *-ose* words: *glucose, sucrose, galactose, maltose, dextrose, fructose*, fats and oils (vegetables oil, soybean oil) or salt. If these ingredients appear near the beginning of the list, the food is likely not a healthy choice. In addition, as a general rule, the shorter the ingredient list, the better. For the most part, you should be able to pronounce and understand every ingredient listed.

APPENDIX 3
THE GLYCEMIC INDEX

The glycemic index is a scale that measures the speed of entry of a carbohydrate food source into the bloodstream. The faster the entry, the more insulin (a fat storage hormone) is secreted in response. All foods are given a value on the glycemic index (GI) according to the extent to which they raise blood sugar levels after being consumed, according to these categories:

- Low-GI food = a value of less than 55
- Medium-GI food = a value from 55 to 70
- High-GI food = a value of more than 70

When a food GI type falls within a range, it's listed by its average. For instance, a banana's GI type depends on ripeness, with the rating ranging from 42 (unripe/low) to 70 (extremely ripe/medium); the average is 54 (low). The glycemic load (GL) takes the serving size (i.e., the number of grams of carbohydrates) into account. The GL is calculated by multiplying the GI by the amount of available carbohydrates in a serving divided by 100. The GL rankings are:

- Low-GL food = a value from 0 to 10
- Medium-GL food = a value from 11 to 19
- High-GL food = a value of 20 or more

Glycemic Index Value and Type of Selected Foods

Food	GI Value	GI Type
Fruits		
Apple	39	Low
Apple juice	40	Low
Apricot	57	Medium
Banana	54	Low
Cantaloupe	65	Medium
Cherries	22	Low
Grapefruit	25	Low
Grapefruit juice	48	Low
Grapes	46	Low
Kiwi	52	Low
Mango	56	Medium
Orange	44	Low
Orange juice	47	Low
Peach	42	Low
Pear	37	Low
Pineapple	66	Medium
Pineapple juice	46	Low
Plum	38	Low
Strawberries	40	Low
Sultana raisins	56	Medium
Watermelon	72	High

Food	GI Value	GI Type
Vegetables		
Artichoke	15	Low
Asparagus	14	Low
Bell pepper	10	Low
Broccoli	10	Low
Brussels sprouts	16	Low
Beet	63	Medium
Cabbage	10	Low
Carrot	70	Medium
Cauliflower	15	Low
Celery	15	Low
Green beans	14	Low
Lettuce	10	Low
Mushrooms	10	Low
Onion	10	Low
Parsnip	98	High
Potato, boiled	56	Medium
Potato, mashed	70	Medium
Potato, baked	84	High
Sweet corn	55	Medium
Sweet potato	50	Low
Yam	50	Low
Legumes		
Baked beans	48	Low
Black-eyed beans	42	Low
Broad beans	79	High
Butter beans	31	Low
Chickpeas	33	Low
Green beans	37	Low

Food	GI Value	GI Type
Haricot (white navy) beans	38	Low
Lentils	25	Low
Lima beans	31	Low
Peanuts	14	Low
Pinto beans	38	Low
Red kidney beans	27	Low
Snap peas	38	Low
Soybeans	18	Low
Split peas	31	Low
Grains, pasta and rice		
Barley	35	Low
Buckwheat	55	Medium
Couscous	65	Medium
Cornmeal	70	Medium
Wheat	48	Low
Rye	35	Low
Millet	70	Medium
Oat bran	54	Low
Pasta, gluten-free	54	Low
Pasta, regular*	49	Low
Capellini	46	Low
Fettuccine	32	Low
Gnocchi	66	Medium
Linguini	52	Low
Macaroni	45	Low
Noodles, instant	46	Low
Noodles, rice	61	Medium
Spaghetti	41	Low
Rice, basmati	58	Medium

Rice, brown	51	Low
Rice, white	72	High
Rice, wild	58	Medium

*Although pasta has a relatively low GI value (anywhere from 30 to 60), this does not mean it is suitable to eat in large quantities for weight loss. Pasta is dense in carbohydrates and should be consumed only in limited amounts. Cook it so it's al dente (firm when bitten) to lower the glycemic index value.

Food	GI Value	GI Type
Milk Products*		
Buttermilk	—	Low
Chocolate milk	34	Low
Custard	43	Low
Goat's milk	—	Low
Ice cream, regular	61	Medium
Ice cream, low-fat	50	Low
Milk, partially skimmed	34	Low
Milk, skimmed	32	Low
Milk, whole	27	Low
Soy milk, flavoured	30	Low
Yogurt, regular, plain	35	Low
Yogurt, low-fat, plain	14	Low
Yogurt, low-fat, sweetened	33	Low
Yogurt, low-fat, non-sweetened	14	Low
Breads and cereals		
Bagel	72	High
Baguette, French	95	Very high
Bread, gluten-free	89	High

* refers to cow's milk, unless otherwise stated

Food	GI Value	GI Type
Bread, high-fibre	68	Medium
Bread, white	71	High
Bread, whole-grain	69	Medium
Crispbread	81	High
Croissant	67	Medium
Crumpet	69	Medium
Doughnut	76	High
Hamburger bun	61	Medium
Linseed rye bread	55	Medium
Pastry	60	Medium
Pita bread	57	Medium
Pizza	60	Medium
Rice cakes	85	High
Rye bread	41	Low
Ryvita	69	Medium
Waffles	75	High
All-Bran (all types)	42	Low
Cheerios	74	High
Coco Pops	77	High
Corn Flakes	84	High
Muesli	56	Medium
Oat bran	55	Medium
Porridge	42	Low
Rice Krispies	82	High
Shredded Wheat	67	Medium
Special K	64	Medium
Sultana Bread	52	Low
Sustain	68	Medium
Wheetabix	69	Medium

Glycemic Load Ratings of Selected Foods

Below 10 = Low; 11 to 19 = medium; above 20 = high

Food	Carbohydrates (grams per serving)	Glycemic Load (per serving)
Fruits		
Apple	21.0	8
Banana	26.5	14
Cantaloupe	13.5	9
Orange	16.0	7
Pineapple	19.0	12
Raisins, 1/2 cup (125 mL)	44.0	28
Watermelon	6.0	4
Vegetables		
Asparagus (6 spears)	4.0	1
Broccoli, steamed, 1/2 cup (125 mL)	2.0	1
Cabbage, raw, 1 cup (250 mL)	7.5	1
Carrots, raw, 1 cup (250 mL)	6.0	3
Corn, 1 cob	29.0	15
French fries, 1/2 cup (125 mL)	29.0	22
Green beans, boiled, 1/2 cup (125 mL)	5.0	1
Green peas, boiled, 1/2 cup (125 mL)	6.0	3
Potato, white, baked	30.5	26
Spinach, steamed, 1/2 cup (125 mL)	3.5	1
Sweet potato	28.0	17
Tomatoes, raw, 1 cup (250 mL)	5.0	1

Food	Carbohydrates (grams per serving)	Glycemic Load (per serving)
Grains		
Bagel, white, 2 oz (60 g)	32.0	23
Bread, white, 1 slice	14.0	10
Bread, whole-grain, 1 slice	14.0	7
Corn tortilla (1)	23.0	12
Hamburger bun (1 avg.)	15.0	9
Pumpernickel bread, 1 slice	15.0	8
Rice, brown, cooked, 1 cup (250 mL)	33.0	18
Rice, white, cooked, 1 cup (250 mL)	40.0	26
Spaghetti, boiled, 1 cup (250 mL)	45.0	27
Waffle, 7-inch (18 cm)	27.0	21
Cereals		
All-Bran, 1 cup (250 mL)	22.0	9
Coco Pops, 1 cup (250 mL)	47.0	36
Corn Flakes, 1 cup (250 mL)	33.0	27
Cream of Wheat, 1 cup (250 mL)	30.0	22
Oatmeal, 1 cup (250 mL)	28	16
Raisin Bran, 1 cup (250 mL)	45.0	27
Special K, 1 cup (250 mL)	36.0	25

Food	Carbohydrates (grams per serving)	Glycemic Load (per serving)
Dairy Products		
Ice cream, 1 cup (250 mL)	13.0	8
Milk, 2%, 1 cup (250 mL)	12.0	4
Yogurt, reduced-fat with fruit	26.0	7
Snack foods		
Apple pie	29.5	13
Banana bread	37.5	18
Cashews, salted, 2 oz (60 g)	13.5	3
Chicken nuggets	15.0	7
Corn chips	27.0	17
Graham crackers	19.0	14
Peanuts, 2 oz (60 g)	10.0	1
Pizza, supreme, 1 slice	25.0	9
Popcorn, microwave, plain	5.0	4
Potato chips	20.0	11
Pretzels	19.0	16
Rice cakes	22.0	17
Snickers bar	34.5	19
Vanilla wafers	18.0	14
Beverages		
Apple juice, 8 oz (250 mL)	30.0	12
Orange juice, 8 oz (250 mL)	26.0	13
Pepsi, 8 oz (250 mL)	35.0	15
Tomato juice, 1/2 cup (125 mL)	10.0	4

Source: Adapted from Kaye Foster-Powell et al, International tables of glycemic index and glycemic load values: *American Journal of Clinical Nutrition*, vol. 76, 2002, pages 5–56.

APPENDIX 4

HEALTHIEST COOKING FATS

The following are healthy fats that are ideal for cooking. When purchasing oils, look for cold expeller-pressed oils that are stored in dark bottles.

Butter

Type of fat: saturated

Butter is a medium-chain fatty acid, like coconut oil, that has received an unfair bad rap. Butter is a great source of fat-soluble vitamins, including vitamins A and D. Again, portion size is important. Butter tends to burn when cooking and is best to cook with at medium heat.

Canola oil

Type of fat: monounsaturated

Canola oil should be purchased organic and expeller pressed when possible. Canola oil is a fairly stable oil that lends a very mild flavour, making it great for any dish.

Coconut oil

Type of fat: saturated

Although coconut oil is a saturated fat, it does not contain any cholesterol and is a healthy medium-chain fatty acid. Medium-chain fatty acids are a great source of energy in the body and are rarely stored as fat. Coconut oil is one of the most stable oils for cooking, with a very high smoke point. As with all oils, portion size is important. One serving of coconut oil is 1 teaspoon (5 mL).

Ghee

Type of fat: saturated

Ghee is a clarified butter that lends a delicious taste to foods. Ghee does not burn as easily as regular butter and can often take the place of oils for cooking. When stir-frying with ghee, you do not need to use as much as if you were cooking as with oil.

Grapeseed oil

Type of fat: polyunsaturated—omega-6

Grapeseed oil has a very mild flavour and is great for cooking. It is a fairly stable oil and can be used for cooking at higher temperatures (e.g., for stir-fries and searing meats).

Olive oil

Type of fat: monounsaturated

Olive oil is a highly nutritious fat. This popular oil is one of the staples in the Mediterranean diet and has been shown to decrease the risk of heart disease and stroke. Olive oil is not ideal for cooking at high heat, as it can decompose under extreme temperatures, causing free radicals and other dangerous molecules to replace the natural antioxidants. When stove-top cooking with olive oil, keep the pan temperature at medium to low heat and watch the temperature during the cooking process. Olive oil is also great for drizzling on whole-grain bread, sautéing vegetables, adding to tomato sauce and in salad dressings.

Sesame oil

Type of fat: polyunsaturated—omega-6

Sesame oil has an intense flavour and is needed only in small amounts to deliver a punch of terrific taste. Sesame oil is great for cooking, as it has a high smoke point. Try using sesame oil in Asian-style dishes such as stir-fries and in soups and marinades.

APPENDIX 5
SUPPLEMENTS

For specific product recommendations, visit www.drjoey.com.

ADRENAL HEALTH

The adrenal glands are a small pair of organs that sit on top of the kidneys. These glands produce the hormones cortisone, cortisol, aldosterone and DHEA. During times of heightened stress, greater demand is placed upon the adrenal glands. If these glands are overtaxed due to prolonged periods of stress, malfunctioning can occur, leading to adrenal fatigue. Supplements to support and protect adrenal health include:

- **B vitamins.** This group of vitamins are like spark plugs to each one of our trillions of cells, promoting optimal energy levels. During times of stress our body uses more B vitamins. Taking a supplement can help prevent deficiency and boost energy levels. When purchasing a B vitamin to lower your stress response and support adrenal function, be sure to purchase a vitamin B complex. For best results, select a multi-B that has 50 milligrams each of the B vitamins.

- **Vitamin C.** Essential for the adrenal glands to function properly. During times of stress we require more vitamin C to regulate adrenal gland function and support our immune system. This is one of the reasons that we tend to get sick more often when we are stressed. During times of heightened stress, vitamin C with bioflavonoids is recommended (3,000 to 5,000 milligrams in divided doses).

- **Rhodiola.** This mighty herb is well known as an adaptogen, which is thought to increase the body's resistance to stress and generally enhance physical and mental functioning. Rhodiola is known to improve energy levels and feelings of well-being during times of increased stress—indeed, it is commonly used by endurance athletes to maintain energy and vitality during such times. The recommended dosage is 100 milligrams standardized extract with a minimum of 3.5% to 4% rosavins and 4.5% salidrosides, taken twice daily. Rhodiola is not recommended for women with a history of breast cancer.

- **Maca.** A Peruvian root known to support our bodies during times of stress by promoting optimal energy levels and hormonal balance.

- **Multivitamin and multimineral complex.** Necessary to support adrenal health. Use a high-potency formula.

- **Chlorophyll.** A natural blood cleanser that can also help to support adrenal health and overall well-being. Add 1 tbsp (5 mL) to water 2 times per day.

- **Greens +.** A high-potency alkaline green powder that can support overall mood and well-being. For more information visit www.drjoey.com.

Other ways to support and protect adrenal health:

- Avoid refined flours, sugars and caffeine.
- Work out moderately.
- Include plenty of cold-water fish, fresh vegetables and colourful fruits in your diet.
- Include nuts and seeds in your diet.
- Practice visualization, yoga, meditation and journaling to help reduce stress.

MENOPAUSE

Certain supplements can be enormously helpful in reducing symptoms associated with menopause, such as hot flashes, moodiness and weight gain around the abdominal region. I have seen women sail through menopause by using the supplements listed here.

- **Flaxseed.** Well known for its high lignan content. Lignans are important for hormone balance and can alleviate many common menopausal symptoms.

- **Organic soy protein.** Soy protein contains phytoestrogens, mild estrogens that can help diminish common menopause complaints, such as hot flashes and night sweats. Enjoying high-quality whole soy foods can also achieve the same results. These foods include miso, tofu and tempeh. (For more on the benefits and drawbacks of soy, see Appendix 1, pages 279–281.)

- **Maca.** An amazing supplement for hormone balance. Maca has been shown to be beneficial for women suffering from menopausal symptoms, especially those with a high-stress lifestyle.

- **Black cohosh, licorice, fennel, anise and soy.** All have been shown to be natural estrogen promoters. Do not take black cohosh if you are pregnant or have liver problems.

- **Calcium with magnesium and vitamin D.** Calcium and magnesium are the two most abundant minerals in the body. Vitamin D is needed for proper absorption of these two key minerals. This is an important supplement to maintain optimal bone health and prevent osteoporosis.

- **Fish oils.** These oils can help with hot flashes and hormonal balance; they are also anti-inflammatory. The recommended dosage is a minimum of 1,000 milligrams 3 times per day. (See Appendix 1, pages 273–274, for more details.)

- **Vitamin B complex.** A powerful anti-stress supplement to help support the adrenal cortex.

CRAVINGS

Cravings are not a sign that you are weak, but rather that your blood sugars are not balanced. The supplements in the following list are very effective at balancing blood sugars and getting rid of cravings once and for all.

- **Chromium.** A key trace mineral in blood sugar metabolism. The suggested dosage is from 200 to 800 micrograms per day. If you are on medication for blood sugar control, talk to your doctor before taking this.

- **5-HTP.** A precursor to serotonin, also known as your "feel good" hormone. Optimal levels of serotonin can help to curb appetite and reduce cravings.

- **High-quality whey protein isolate.** Mix this powder with water or almond milk and take between meals to help balance blood sugar levels and reduce sugar cravings.

BOOSTING METABOLISM

- **Chromium.** An essential mineral for blood sugar balance. Studies show that it can also help boost weight loss results.

- **CLA, or conjugated linoleic acid.** A type of fatty acid that has been studied and shown to help your body use your fat stores more efficiently. CLA is known to help in the reduction of body fat in the midsection (abdominal region). It also improves insulin sensitivity, thereby decreasing insulin and decreasing fat storage.

- **Green tea.** The phytonutrients in green tea are well-known antioxidants that promote weight loss by causing a thermogenic effect in the body that boosts metabolism. The increased heat in the body burns calories.

- **High-quality whey protein isolate powder.** High-quality protein is an essential in any weight loss program. Whey protein isolate is a great source of easy-to-digest protein. It boosts metabolism by keeping blood sugars balanced, maintains metabolically active muscle tissue and helps to reduce cravings.

- **Fish oils.** Many people are afraid of fat when it comes to weight loss; however, fat is essential for healthy weight loss. Fish oil contains omega-3, which helps burn fat. (See Appendix 1, pages 277–279, for more details.)

OPTIMAL HEALTH AND WELL-BEING

- **Fish oils.** Omega-3 fats are the star in fish oils. These fats are essential in our diet and needed for optimal blood sugar control, cardiovascular health and brain health, among other things.

- **Multivitamin and multimineral complex.** A health insurance plan to make sure you are getting a base amount of all essential vitamins and minerals needed to maintain health.

- **Vitamin D.** Studies are now proving more and more the health benefits of this fat-soluble vitamin. Many North Americans are deficient in vitamin D, especially during the winter months. Vitamin D is known as the sunshine vitamin, as we can get our supply directly from the sunshine. If you are not exposed to at least 15 minutes of sunshine per day (without sunscreen), you may want to consider a supplement.

- **Probiotics.** These healthy bacteria are essential for overall health. When these good bacteria enter our intestinal track they provide optimal digestion, absorption of nutrients and a strong immune system.

APPENDIX 6 - ACID VERSUS ALKALINE FOODS

FOODS	High Acid	Medium Acid	Low Acid	Low Alkaline	Medium Alkaline	High Alkaline
Vegetables, beans, legumes	processed soybeans, salted and sweetened peanut butter	salted and unsweetened peanut butter	corn, lentils, peanuts with skin, organic peanut butter, soy protein powder, beans (kidney, lima, navy, pinto, white, black), peas (green, split, chick), extra-firm tofu, edamame	Brussels sprouts, beets (tops and roots), tomatoes and tomato juice, fresh peas, dark lettuce, all mushrooms, potatoes with skin, pumpkin, squash, tempeh	bell pepper, cauliflower, parsnip, endive, ginger root, sweet potato, cabbage, celery, carrots, asparagus	broccoli, cucumber, cilantro, garlic, oriental greens, onions, kale, spinach, parsley, sea vegetables, Greens +
Fruits	cranberries, dried fruit (sulfured)	prunes, olives, pickles, sweetened fruit juice, canned fruit, jams or preserves	dried fruit, natural figs, dates, bananas, unsweetened canned fruit, natural fruit juice, unsweetened jams and preserves	fresh pineapples, apricots, grapes, blueberries, strawberries, blackberries, papayas	apples, avocados, pink grapefruits, lemons, limes, mangoes, pears, peaches	cantaloupes, honeydews, raisins, nectarines, raspberries, watermelons, fresh black cherries, black olives in oil
Seasonings, herbs, spices	black pepper, MSG, soy sauce, brewer's and nutritional yeast	vanilla, nutmeg, mayonnaise, ketchup	tahini, carob, cocoa, regular table salt	most herbs, curry, mustard powder, kola nut, tamari, milk thistle, maca, astragalus, suma, echinacea	cinnamon, ginger, dill, mint, peppermint, turmeric, rhodiola, basil, oregano, licorice root, Siberian ginseng	Celtic sea salt, Real Salt (Great Salt Lake), miso and natto, cayenne, ashwagandha, gotu kola, ginkgo biloba, baking soda (sodium bicarbonate)
Beverages	alcoholic drinks, soft drinks	coffee (milk and sugar)	unsweetened soy milk and rice milk, black tea, black and decaf coffee	dry red wine, unsweetened almond milk, distilled water, beer (draft) or dark stout, black coffee (organic)	teas (green, matcha green, ginger, rooibos, chamomile), water, ozonoated water, ionized water, aloe vera juice	electron-rich alkaline water, plasma-activated water (PAW), Greens +
Grains, cereals, other	barley, pastries, cakes, tarts, cookies	plain rice protein powder, rolled oats and oat bran, rye, white bread, white pasta, white rice	brown and basmati rice, wheat, buckwheat, kasha, amaranth, whole wheat and corn pasta, whole grain bread	whole oats, quinoa, wild rice, millet, spelt, hemp protein powder		bee pollen, soy lecithin granules, dairy-free probiotic cultures
Nuts, seeds, grasses, sprouts, oils	pistachios, trans fatty acids, acrylamides	cashews, pecans, walnuts	popcorn, canola oil, grapeseed oil, green soybeans, pine nuts, safflower oil	hazelnuts, flaxseed and sea buckthorn oils, hemp seeds and oil, sesame seeds and oil, sunflower seeds and oil, fresh coconut and oil	extra-virgin olive oil, borage and primrose oil, chestnuts, Brazil nuts, light and dark flaxseeds, macadamia nuts, black currant oil	pumpkin seeds, almonds with skin, plain almond butter with skin, all sprouts, wheat grass, alfalfa grass, barley grass
Meats, fish, poultry	beef, lobster	chicken, lamb, pork, veal	fish, turkey, venison, wild duck, seafood	cod liver oil	wild and pure omega-3 fish oil, CLA (conjugated linoleic acid)	
Dairy, eggs	processed cheese, hard cheese, egg yolks (chicken)	soy cheese and soft cheese, ice cream, whole eggs (chicken)	cow's milk, cream, yogurt, butter, buttermilk, egg whites (chicken)	soft goat cheese, fresh goat milk	dairy probiotic cultures, whey protein isolate powder	human breast milk
Sweeteners	artificial sweeteners	corn syrup and fructose, high-fructose corn syrup, sugar	commercial honey	stevia, brown rice syrup, pure maple syrup, unpasteurized honey	blackstrap molasses (unsulphured)	
Vinegar	white vinegar	balsamic vinegar	rice vinegar		apple cider vinegar	

Source: Adapted from material created by genuinehealth.com.

REFERENCES

Chapter 4

Baer, DJ, et al. Dietary fatty acids affect plasma markers of inflammation in healthy men fed controlled diets: a randomized crossover study. *American Journal of Clinical Nutrition*, 2004, 79(6):969–73.

Gunnarsdottir, I, et al. Inclusion of fish or fish oil in weight-loss diets for young adults: effects on blood lipids. *International Journal of Obesity*, July 2008, 32:1105–12.

Hofmann, S, and M Tschop. Dietary sugars: a fat difference. *Journal of Clinical Investigation*, 2009, 119(5):1089–92.

Steinberger, J, A Moran, CP Hong, DR Jacobs and AR Sinaiko. Adiposity in childhood predicts obesity and insulin resistance in young adulthood. *Journal of Pediatrics*, 2001, 138(4):469–73.

Warren, JM, CJ Henry and V Simonite. Low glycemic index breakfasts and reduced food intake in preadolescent children. *Pediatrics*, 2003, 112(5):e414.

Chapter 5

Herriot, AM, S Whitcroft and Y Jeanes. A retrospective audit of patients with polycystic ovary syndrome: the effects of a reduced glycaemic load diet. *Journal of Human Nutrition and Dietetics*, 2008, 21(4):337–45.

Kasim-Karakas, SE, RU Almario and W Cunningham. Effects of protein versus simple sugar intake on weight loss in polycystic ovary syndrome (according to the National Institutes of Health criteria). *Fertility and Sterility*, 2009, 92:262–70.

Knowler, WC, E Barrett-Connor, SE Fowler, RF Hamman, JM Lachin, EA Walker and DM Nathan. Reduction in the incidence of type 2 diabetes with lifestyle intervention or metformin. *New England Journal of Medicine*, 2002, 346:393–403.

Mavropoulos, JC, WS Yancy, J Hepburn and EC Westman. The effects of a low-carbohydrate, ketogenic diet on the polycystic ovary syndrome: a pilot study. *Nutrition and Metabolism*, 16 December 2005:2–35.

Riccardi, G, and R Giacco. Dietary fat, insulin sensitivity and the metabolic syndrome. *Clinical Nutrition*, 2004, 23:447–56.

Vessby, B, et al. Substituting dietary saturated for monounsaturated fat impairs insulin sensitivity in healthy men and women: the KANWU study. *Diabetologia*, 2001, 44(3):312–29.

Chapter 6

Kaunitz, H, and CS Dayrit. Coconut oil consumption and coronary heart disease. *Philippine Journal of Internal Medicine*, 1992, 30:165–71.

Kurup, PA, and T Rajmohan II. Consumption of coconut oil and coconut kernel and the incidence of atherosclerosis. Coconut and Coconut Oil in Human Nutrition, *Proceedings: Symposium on Coconut and Coconut Oil in Human Nutrition.* (27 March 1994.) Kochi, India: Coconut Development Board, 1995, 35–59.

Prior, IA, F Davidson, CE Salmond and Z Czochanska. Cholesterol, coconuts, and diet on Polynesian atolls: a natural experiment: the Pukapuka and Tokelau Island studies. *American Journal of Clinical Nutrition*, 1981, 34:1552–61.

Chapter 8

DeNoon, DJ. Drink more diet soda, gain more weight? Overweight risk soars 41% with each daily can of diet soft drink. WebMD, 13 June 2005. http://www.webmd.com/diet/news/20050613/drink-more-diet-soda-gain-more-weight.

Siler, SQ, RA Neese and MK Hellerstein. De novo lipogenesis, lipid kinetics, and whole-body lipid balances in humans after acute alcohol consumption. *American Journal of Clinical Nutrition*, 1999, 70:928–36.

Swithers, SE, and TL Davidson. A role for sweet taste: calorie predictive relations in energy regulation by rats. *Behavioral Neuroscience*, 2008, 122(1):161–73.

Chapter 10

American Thoracic Society, international conference, San Diego, 19–24 May 2006, news release.

Arjmandi, BH, and BJ Smith. Soy isoflavones' osteoprotective role in postmenopausal women: mechanism of action. *Journal of Nutritional Biochemistry*, 2002, 13:130–37.

Health Canada. It's your health: food allergies: http://www.hc-sc.gc.ca/hl-vs/iyh-vsv/food-aliment/allerg-eng.php.

Chavarro, JE, TL Toth, SM Sadio and R Hauser. Soy food and isoflavone intake in relation to semen quality parameters among men from an infertility clinic. *Human Reproduction*, 2008, 23:2584–90.

Hamilton-Reeves, JM, G Vazquez, SJ Duval, WR Phipps, MS Kurzer and MJ Messina. Clinical studies show no effects of soy protein or isoflavones on reproductive hormones in men: results of a meta-analysis. *Fertility and Sterility*, Zolo, 94(3):997–1007.

Messina, M, and S Barnes. The role of soy products in reducing risk of cancer. *Journal of the National Cancer Institute*, 1991, 83:541–46.

Messina, MJ, and CL Loprinzi. Soy for breast cancer survivors: a critical review of the literature. *Journal of Nutrition*, 2001, 131:3095S–108S.

Messina, MJ, V Persky, KD Setchell and S Barnes. Soy intake and cancer risk: a review of the in vitro and in vivo data. *Nutrition and Cancer*, 1994, 21:113–31.

Patel, SR, A Malhotra, DP White, DJ Gottlieb and FB Hu. Association between reduced sleep and weight gain in women. *American Journal of Epidemiology*, 2006, 164(10):947–54.

Robbins, J. Tools, resources, and inspiration: what about soy? http://www.johnrobbins.info/blog/what-about-soy/.

Shu, XO, F Jin, Q Dai et al. Soyfood intake during adolescence and subsequent risk of breast cancer among Chinese women. *Cancer Epidemiology, Biomarkers and Prevention*, 2001, 10:483–88.

Trock, BJ, L Hilakivi-Clarke and R Clarke. Meta-analysis of soy intake and breast cancer risk. *Journal of the National Cancer Institute*, 2006, 98:459–71.

US Food and Drug Administration. Food labeling, health claims, soy protein, and coronary heart disease. *Federal Register* 1999, 57:699–733.

Wu, AH, MC Yu, C-C Treng and MC Pike. Epidemiology of soy exposures and breast cancer risk. *British Journal of Cancer*, 2008, 98:9–14.

Yan, L, and E Spitznagel. A meta-analysis of soy foods and risk of breast cancer in women. *International Journal of Cancer Prevention*, 2005, 1:281–93.

Zhaoping, L, et al. Pistachio nuts reduce triglycerides and body weight by comparison to refined carbohydrate snack in obese subjects on a 12-week weight loss program. *Journal of the American College of Nutrition*, 2010, 29(3):198–203.

Appendix

Crawford, V, et al. Effects of niacin-bound chromium supplementation on body composition in overweight African-American women. *Diabetes, Obesity and Metabolism*, 1999, 1:331–37.

Docherty, JP, et al. A double-blind, placebo-controlled, exploratory trial of chromium picolinate in atypical depression: effect on carbohydrate craving. *Journal of Psychiatric Practice*, 2005, 11(5):302–14.

Schanfarber, L. Hormone helpers. alive, http://www.alive.com/3234a6a2.php?subject_bread_cramb=150.

Anton, SD, et al. Effects on chromium picolinate on food intake and satiety. *Diabetes Technology and Therapeutics*, 2008, 10 (5): 405–12.

INDEX